DIABETIC DIET COOKBOOK FOR BEGINNERS AFTER 50

A Guide to Prediabetes & Type 2 Diabetes with Super-Easy, Delicious Days of Low-Sugar & Low-Carb Recipes. Includes 14-Day Meal Plan for a Healthy Lifestyle

Theresa R. Grace

Table Of Contents

INTRODUCTION

Greetings from a journey of sustenance, wellness, and gastronomic delight to you, dear reader! This is a compassionate guide created especially for people navigating the waters of diabetes over 50 years of age, not just a cookbook. Whether you've been managing diabetes for years or you were just recently diagnosed, this book intends to become your go-to kitchen buddy, changing the way you think about food, cooking, and your overall health.

Our bodies change as we get older, and these changes present both new possibilities and challenges. Although managing diabetes might occasionally feel overwhelming, it's critical to keep in mind that you have daily decisions that affect your health. And what better place to start than with the food you consume?

For many people, cooking is a loving act that nourishes the body and the spirit. However, some people may find the thought of adjusting to a "diabetic diet" intimidating, constrictive, or even depressing. But do not worry! With this cookbook, I hope to dispel those myths and demonstrate to you that eating well for diabetes can be fascinating, tasty, and very fulfilling.

Imagine waking up to a meal that tantalizes your taste buds and controls your blood sugar. Imagine a meal that fills you up, gives you energy, and makes you happy—all without raising your blood sugar levels. This cookbook is full of expertly prepared recipes that are meant to make every meal a celebration of flavor and health.

Individuals over 50 have distinct and complex nutritional needs. We frequently experience different health situations that necessitate us to be more attentive to what we consume, and our metabolism slows down and our muscle mass declines. This complexity is further compounded by managing diabetes, but it also presents an opportunity to adopt a diet that promotes general wellness.

Understanding is the first step toward empowerment, and this book seeks to provide you with the information you need to make wise decisions. We'll cover the fundamentals of macronutrients and the glycemic index, as well as the value of portion management and reading food labels, to give you the knowledge you need to make informed dietary decisions.

Having the correct ingredients and tools is the first step toward culinary success. I'll walk you through stocking a diabetes-friendly pantry, selecting necessary kitchen tools, and even meal planning so you're always ready to whip up a tasty and nutritious dinner.

I have personally witnessed the transformational potential of food. More importantly, though, I am aware of the emotional roller coaster that comes with eating adjustments, having assisted family members in managing their diabetes. This cookbook is full of anecdotes, useful advice, and a kind mindset that celebrates the small wins and respects the difficulties.

Every recipe in this book is a step on a gastronomic journey, ranging from filling main courses and sweet desserts to robust breakfasts and cool smoothies. A journey where managing your diabetes and enjoying your meals don't have to be mutually exclusive. Instead, health and flavor go hand in hand.

Now let's set off on this adventure together. Together, we may rediscover the delight of cooking, the satisfaction of eating, and the calm that accompanies taking proactive measures to improve your health. One delicious meal at a time, here's to a new chapter full of flavorful discoveries, vigorous health, and a life well-lived.

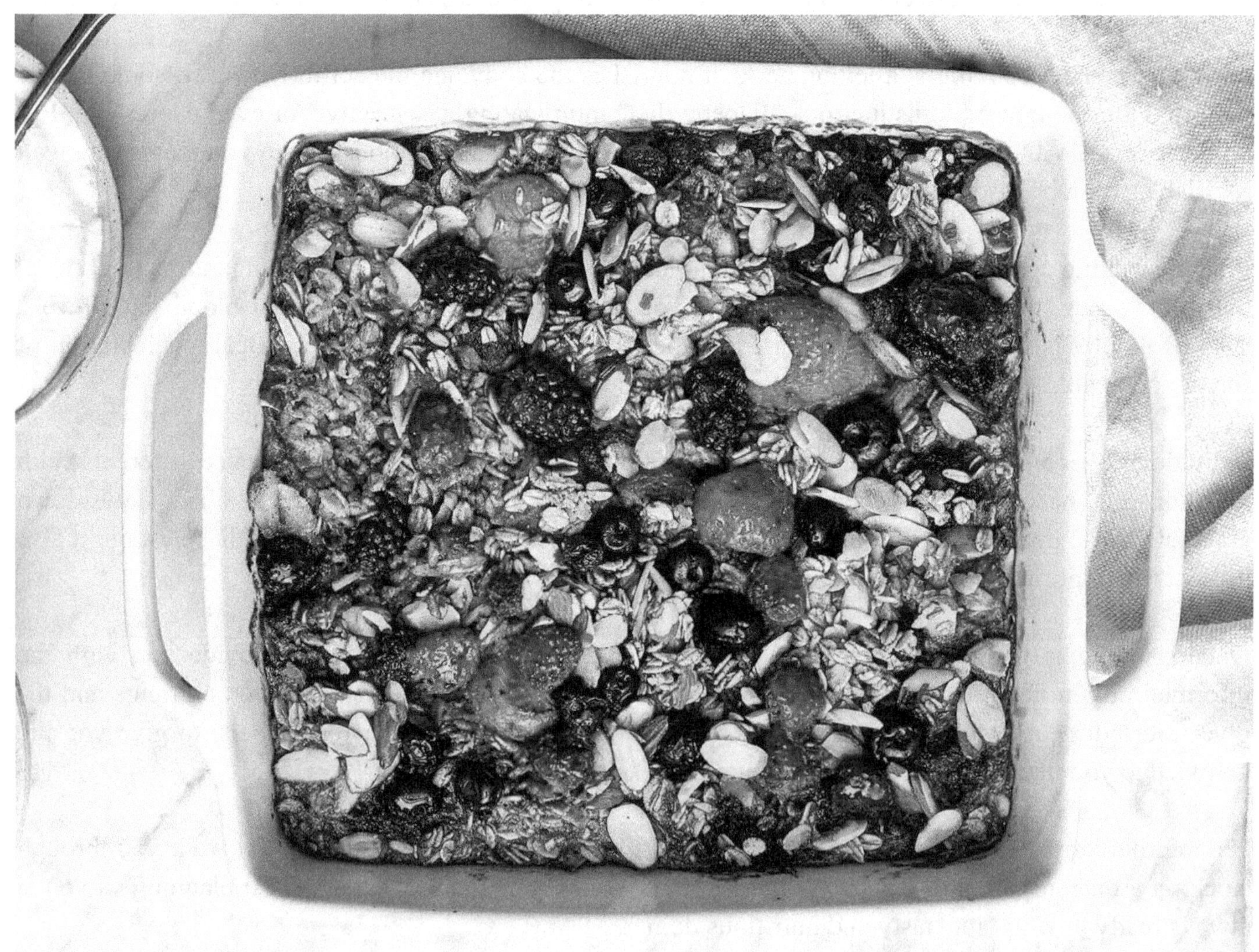

UNDERSTANDING
DIABETES

Diabetes is a long-term medical illness that impacts the body's ability to use food as fuel. It involves insulin, which helps glucose from food enter cells for fuel. When you have diabetes, your body is either unable to use the insulin it produces effectively or is unable to produce enough of it. Too much blood sugar remains in your circulation when there is insufficient insulin or when cells cease reacting to insulin. That can eventually lead to major health issues like renal disease, heart disease, and eyesight loss.

Diabetes can be generally classified into multiple categories, each with unique causes, traits, and therapeutic approaches. Anyone with diabetes must understand these types, but people over 50 should especially understand them because their age raises the risk of complications. Let's examine the many forms of diabetes, their etiology, signs, and bodily effects.

TYPES OF DIABETES

Type 1 Diabetes

Type 1 diabetes is an autoimmune condition where the body attacks the insulin-producing beta cells in the pancreas. This results in little to no insulin production. It was previously known as juvenile diabetes or insulin-dependent diabetes because it typically appears in children and young adults, though it can occur at any age.

Causes

The exact cause of Type 1 diabetes is not entirely understood, but it's believed to be a combination of genetic predisposition and environmental factors. The body's immune system mistakenly targets and destroys the beta cells in the pancreas, which are responsible for producing insulin.

Symptoms

- Frequent urination
- Excessive thirst
- Extreme hunger
- Unintended weight loss
- Fatigue and weakness
- Blurred vision
- Irritability and mood changes
- Bed-wetting in children who previously didn't wet the bed during the night

Management

Managing Type 1 diabetes involves lifelong insulin therapy, as the body can no longer produce insulin. This can be administered through multiple daily injections or an insulin pump. Monitoring blood sugar levels regularly, following a healthy diet, and maintaining physical activity are also crucial components of management.

Type 2 Diabetes

Type 2 diabetes is the most common form of diabetes, accounting for about 90-95% of all cases. It occurs when the body becomes resistant to insulin or when the pancreas cannot produce enough insulin. Unlike Type 1 diabetes, Type 2 diabetes is largely influenced by lifestyle factors and tends to develop later in life, making it more prevalent in adults over 50.

Causes

The primary causes of Type 2 diabetes include genetic factors, obesity, physical inactivity, and poor diet. Family history and ethnicity also play significant roles. Over time, factors such as a high-calorie diet, sedentary lifestyle, and excess body weight, particularly around the abdomen, can lead to insulin resistance.

Symptoms

- Increased thirst and frequent urination
- Increased hunger
- Unintended weight loss
- Fatigue
- Blurred vision
- Slow-healing sores or frequent infections
- Areas of darkened skin, usually in the armpits and neck

Management

Management of Type 2 diabetes often begins with lifestyle changes, such as adopting a healthy diet and increasing physical activity. Weight loss can improve insulin sensitivity. Medications are also used to manage blood sugar levels, and in some cases, insulin therapy may be necessary. Regular monitoring of blood sugar levels is crucial to ensure effective management.

Gestational Diabetes

Gestational diabetes is a type of diabetes that develops during pregnancy and usually goes away after the baby is born. It occurs when the body cannot produce enough insulin to meet the extra needs during pregnancy, leading to high blood sugar levels.

Causes

Hormonal changes during pregnancy can make cells less responsive to insulin, a condition known as insulin resistance. If the pancreas can't produce enough insulin to overcome this resistance, blood sugar levels rise, resulting in gestational diabetes. Risk factors include being overweight, having a family history of diabetes, and being older than 25 during pregnancy.

Symptoms

Gestational diabetes often has no noticeable symptoms, which is why regular screening during pregnancy is important. Some symptoms may include:

- Increased thirst
- Frequent urination
- Fatigue
- Nausea

Management

Managing gestational diabetes involves monitoring blood sugar levels, following a healthy diet, exercising regularly, and sometimes taking insulin or oral medications. Proper management is essential to prevent complications for both the mother and the baby.

Prediabetes

Prediabetes is a condition where blood sugar levels are higher than normal but not high enough to be classified as Type 2 diabetes. It is a critical warning sign that indicates an increased risk of developing Type 2 diabetes, heart disease, and stroke.

Causes

The causes of prediabetes are similar to those of Type 2 diabetes and include genetic predisposition, obesity, and a sedentary lifestyle. Insulin resistance plays a significant role, where the body's cells don't respond to insulin effectively.

Symptoms

Prediabetes usually has no clear symptoms, but some individuals might experience symptoms similar to those of diabetes, such as increased thirst and frequent urination. Acanthosis nigricans, a condition characterized by darkened skin in certain areas, can also be a sign of insulin resistance.

Management

Early intervention is key to preventing the progression from prediabetes to Type 2 diabetes. Management strategies include:

- Losing weight
- Eating a healthy diet rich in whole foods, and fiber, and low in sugars and refined carbohydrates
- Increasing physical activity
- Regular monitoring of blood sugar levels

SPECIFIC TYPES OF DIABETES

Maturity Onset Diabetes of the Young (MODY)

MODY is a rare form of diabetes caused by a mutation in a single gene. It often develops in adolescence or early adulthood and is sometimes misdiagnosed as Type 1 or Type 2 diabetes. Management depends on the specific gene affected but can include dietary changes, oral medications, and in some cases, insulin.

Latent Autoimmune Diabetes in Adults (LADA)

LADA is a slow-progressing form of autoimmune diabetes that is often diagnosed in adults over 30. It shares characteristics of both Type 1 and Type 2 diabetes. Initially, it may not require insulin, but over time, the need for insulin therapy becomes necessary. LADA can be misdiagnosed as Type 2 diabetes due to its slower progression and later onset.

Secondary Diabetes

Secondary diabetes results from another medical condition or treatment, such as cystic fibrosis, pancreatitis, or the use of certain medications like glucocorticoids. Management focuses on treating the underlying condition while also controlling blood sugar levels.

Impact of Age on Diabetes

For individuals over 50, managing diabetes requires special considerations due to age-related changes in the body and the increased risk of complications. Aging can affect insulin production and sensitivity, and older adults may have additional health concerns that complicate diabetes management. Here are some factors to consider:

Complications and Risks

- **Cardiovascular Disease**: Diabetes significantly increases the risk of heart disease and stroke, particularly in older adults.
- **Kidney Disease**: Diabetes is a leading cause of chronic kidney disease and kidney failure.
- **Vision Problems**: Diabetic retinopathy, cataracts, and glaucoma are common complications that can impair vision.
- **Nerve Damage**: Peripheral neuropathy, causing pain or loss of sensation in the extremities, is a common issue.
- **Foot Problems**: Poor circulation and nerve damage can lead to foot ulcers and infections.

Management Considerations

- **Comprehensive Care**: Regular check-ups with healthcare providers, including endocrinologists, cardiologists, and ophthalmologists, are essential.
- **Medication Management**: As the body changes with age, medication dosages and types may need adjustment. It's important to review medications regularly with a healthcare provider.
- **Diet and Exercise**: Adopting a balanced diet rich in nutrients and engaging in regular physical activity are crucial. Weight management becomes more important to improve insulin sensitivity and overall health.
- **Monitoring**: Regular monitoring of blood sugar levels, blood pressure, and cholesterol is critical to managing diabetes effectively and preventing complications.

Understanding the different types of diabetes is crucial for effective management and prevention. Each type has unique causes, symptoms, and treatment strategies, but the goal remains the same: to maintain healthy blood sugar levels and prevent complications. For those over 50, managing diabetes involves additional considerations due to the increased risk of complications and the natural changes that come with aging. By staying informed, adopting a healthy lifestyle, and working closely with healthcare providers, individuals with diabetes can lead healthy, fulfilling lives.

IMPORTANCE OF DIET IN MANAGING DIABETES

A chronic illness defined by high blood sugar (glucose) levels, diabetes affects millions of individuals globally. To avoid problems including heart disease, kidney failure, neuropathy, and visual loss, it is imperative to control it. Although insulin therapy and medicine are important tools for regulating blood sugar, food is still the most important aspect of managing diabetes. The relevance of food increases significantly for people over 50 because of the normal metabolic changes that come with age. We will explore the fundamentals of a diabetic-friendly diet, the reasons why diet is important for managing diabetes, and helpful hints for making dietary adjustments in this in-depth investigation.

Blood Sugar and Diabetes

It is crucial to comprehend how the body handles sugar if one is to appreciate the role nutrition plays in the control of diabetes. Upon consumption, the bloodstream is supplied with glucose, which is produced when the carbs in our food are broken down. Insulin, a hormone that aids cells in absorbing glucose for energy, is released by the pancreas in response. This process is compromised in diabetics. Type 2 diabetes is characterized by insulin resistance, in which cells fail to respond to insulin as they should. Type 1 diabetes is characterized by the body's inability to create insulin.

The Role of Diet in Blood Sugar Control

Diet directly influences blood sugar levels. By carefully selecting what and when to eat, individuals with diabetes can maintain more stable blood glucose levels. Here are key ways diet impacts diabetes management:

1. Carbohydrate Control

Carbohydrates have the most immediate effect on blood sugar levels. When digested, they are converted into glucose. The amount and type of carbohydrates consumed can cause significant fluctuations in blood sugar levels. For diabetics, it's crucial to monitor carbohydrate intake and choose complex carbohydrates over simple ones.

- **Simple Carbohydrates**: Found in sugary foods and drinks, they cause rapid spikes in blood sugar.
- **Complex Carbohydrates**: Found in whole grains, vegetables, and legumes, they are digested more slowly, leading to a gradual increase in blood sugar.

Counting carbohydrates and spreading their intake throughout the day helps in preventing blood sugar spikes.

2. Glycemic Index (GI)

The glycemic index measures how quickly a carbohydrate-containing food raises blood sugar levels. Foods with a low GI are digested and absorbed more slowly, causing a gradual rise in blood sugar, while high GI foods cause quick spikes.

- **Low GI Foods**: Whole grains, legumes, non-starchy vegetables, most fruits.
- **High GI Foods**: White bread, sugary cereals, baked goods, and many processed foods.

Diabetics should prioritize low GI foods to maintain stable blood sugar levels.

3. Fiber Intake

Fiber, particularly soluble fiber, slows down the digestion and absorption of carbohydrates, leading to more gradual increases in blood sugar levels. High-fiber foods also promote a feeling of fullness, which can help with weight management—a crucial factor in managing Type 2 diabetes.

- **High-Fiber Foods**: Whole grains, fruits, vegetables, legumes, nuts, and seeds.

4. Protein and Healthy Fats

Including adequate protein and healthy fats in meals can stabilize blood sugar levels by slowing down the absorption of carbohydrates.

- **Proteins**: Lean meats, fish, eggs, dairy, tofu, legumes.
- **Healthy Fats**: Avocado, nuts, seeds, olive oil, fatty fish.

5. Portion Control

Overeating, even healthy foods, can lead to elevated blood sugar levels. Understanding portion sizes and eating moderate amounts at regular intervals helps in maintaining consistent blood sugar levels.

The Impact of Diet on Long-Term Health

Beyond immediate blood sugar control, a well-managed diet has significant long-term benefits for individuals with diabetes:

1. Cardiovascular Health

Diabetes significantly increases the risk of cardiovascular disease. A diet low in saturated fats, trans fats, cholesterol, and sodium can help manage blood pressure and cholesterol levels, reducing the risk of heart disease and stroke.

- **Heart-Healthy Choices**: Fish, especially those rich in omega-3 fatty acids (like salmon and mackerel), nuts, seeds, olive oil, and plenty of fruits and vegetables.

2. Weight Management

Excess body weight, particularly around the abdomen, is a major risk factor for Type 2 diabetes. Weight loss through a balanced diet and regular physical activity improves insulin sensitivity and blood sugar control.

- **Weight-Friendly Foods**: High-fiber foods, lean proteins, and low-calorie vegetables.

3. Kidney Health

Diabetes is a leading cause of kidney disease. Controlling blood sugar and blood pressure through diet can prevent or delay kidney damage.

- **Kidney-Friendly Choices**: Foods low in sodium and phosphorus, and adequate fluid intake.

4. Nerve and Eye Health

Consistently high blood sugar levels can damage nerves and blood vessels in the eyes. A healthy diet that controls blood sugar levels helps prevent diabetic neuropathy and retinopathy.

Tips for Implementing a Diabetic Diet

Implementing dietary changes can be challenging, especially for those over 50 who may have established eating habits. Here are practical tips to help transition to a diabetic-friendly diet:

1. **Plan your Meals:** Planning meals ahead of time ensures that you include a variety of nutrients and avoid last-minute unhealthy choices. Use tools like meal planners or apps to track your food intake and ensure balanced meals.
2. **Cook at Home:** Cooking at home allows you to control the ingredients and cooking methods, reducing the intake of unhealthy fats, sugars, and sodium. Explore diabetic-friendly recipes that are simple and flavorful.
3. **Read Food Labels:** Learning to read and understand food labels helps you make informed choices. Look for the carbohydrate content, added sugars, fiber, and serving size. Avoid products with high levels of added sugars and unhealthy fats.
4. **Incorporate More Vegetables:** Vegetables are low in calories and high in fiber, vitamins, and minerals. Aim to fill half your plate with non-starchy vegetables at each meal. Experiment with different ways of preparing vegetables to keep meals interesting.
5. **Choose Whole Grains:** Replace refined grains with whole grains. Whole grains have more fiber and nutrients, and they have a lower glycemic index. Examples include brown rice, quinoa, barley, and whole wheat products.
6. **Be Mindful of Fruit Intake:** While fruits are healthy, they contain natural sugars. Opt for low-GI fruits and monitor portions. Berries, apples, and pears are good choices.
7. **Limit Sugary Drinks:** Sugary drinks can cause rapid spikes in blood sugar levels. Replace them with water, unsweetened tea, or sparkling water with a splash of lemon or lime.
8. **Snack Wisely:** Choose snacks that combine protein, fiber, and healthy fats to maintain blood sugar levels. Examples include a handful of nuts, yogurt with berries, or hummus with vegetable sticks.

Diet plays an indispensable role in managing diabetes, particularly for individuals over 50 who may face additional health challenges. By focusing on balanced, nutrient-rich meals that control carbohydrate intake and prioritize low-glycemic foods, those with diabetes can achieve better blood sugar control and reduce the risk of complications. The principles of a diabetic-friendly diet—monitoring carbohydrates, incorporating fiber, choosing healthy proteins and fats, and practicing portion control—form the foundation of effective diabetes management.

Moreover, adopting these dietary habits contributes to overall health, promoting cardiovascular health, supporting weight management, protecting kidney function, and preserving nerve and eye health. With careful planning, informed choices, and a commitment to healthy eating, managing diabetes through diet becomes a sustainable and empowering approach, improving quality of life and health outcomes for those over 50.

NUTRITION BASICS FOR DIABETICS OVER 50

MACRONUTRIENTS AND MICRONUTRIENTS

Macronutrients are the nutrients we need in larger quantities to provide energy and maintain body functions. They include carbohydrates, proteins, and fats. Each plays a unique role in our health, and understanding these roles is vital for managing diabetes, especially as we age.

Carbohydrates: Not All Are Created Equal

Carbohydrates are often viewed with suspicion in diabetic diets, but they are an essential part of a balanced diet. The key is to focus on the right types of carbohydrates and control portion sizes.

Simple vs. Complex Carbohydrates

- **Simple Carbohydrates**: These are found in sugars, honey, and many processed foods. They are quickly absorbed into the bloodstream, causing rapid spikes in blood sugar levels. Foods high in simple carbs include candy, soda, and baked goods made with white flour. For diabetics, especially those over 50, it's crucial to limit these foods.
- **Complex Carbohydrates**: These are found in whole grains, legumes, vegetables, and fruits. They take longer to digest, resulting in a more gradual release of glucose into the bloodstream. This helps maintain stable blood sugar levels. Examples include oatmeal, brown rice, quinoa, lentils, and whole-wheat bread.

Fiber: Your Blood Sugar's Best Friend

Dietary fiber, a type of carbohydrate, is particularly beneficial for diabetics. It's not digested or absorbed by the body, so it doesn't raise blood sugar levels. Fiber comes in two forms:

- **Soluble Fiber**: Found in oats, apples, and beans, soluble fiber dissolves in water to form a gel-like substance. It can help lower blood sugar levels by slowing down the absorption of sugar.
- **Insoluble Fiber**: Found in whole grains, nuts, and many vegetables, insoluble fiber helps with digestion and prevents constipation. It doesn't directly affect blood sugar but promotes overall digestive health.

Glycemic Index and Glycemic Load

Understanding the glycemic index (GI) and glycemic load (GL) can help manage blood sugar levels. The GI ranks carbohydrates on a scale from 0 to 100 based on how quickly they raise blood sugar levels. Foods with a high GI cause rapid spikes, while those with a low GI lead to a slower increase.

- **Low GI Foods**: Whole grains, legumes, most fruits, and non-starchy vegetables.
- **High GI Foods**: White bread, rice, and many processed foods.

Glycemic load takes into account the GI and the amount of carbohydrate in a serving, providing a more accurate picture of a food's impact on blood sugar.

Portion Control and Timing

Managing portions is critical. Even healthy carbohydrates can affect blood sugar if eaten in large quantities. Spreading carbohydrate intake throughout the day by eating smaller, more frequent meals can help keep blood sugar levels stable.

Proteins: The Body's Repair Crew

Proteins are vital for maintaining muscle mass, repairing tissues, and supporting the immune system. As we age, muscle mass naturally decreases, making protein even more essential.

Sources of Protein

- **Animal Proteins**: Lean meats (chicken, turkey), fish, eggs, and dairy products (low-fat yogurt, milk). These are complete proteins, meaning they contain all essential amino acids.
- **Plant Proteins**: Beans, lentils, tofu, tempeh, nuts, and seeds. While many plant proteins are not complete, combining different sources (like beans and rice) can provide all essential amino acids.

Portion Sizes and Protein Balance

Balancing protein with other macronutrients is important. A typical serving size of protein should be about the size of your palm. Overconsumption can lead to increased fat intake, especially if proteins come from fatty meats or full-fat dairy products.

Benefits of Protein for Diabetics Over 50

- **Blood Sugar Control**: Protein doesn't raise blood sugar levels as carbohydrates do. Including a source of protein with each meal can help stabilize blood sugar.
- **Muscle Maintenance**: Adequate protein intake helps preserve muscle mass, which is important for overall health and mobility.

Fats: The Essential Energy Source

Fats are essential for absorbing vitamins, protecting organs, and providing long-lasting energy. However, not all fats are created equal.

Types of Fats

- **Unsaturated Fats**: These are the healthy fats found in olive oil, avocados, nuts, and fatty fish (like salmon). They can improve heart health and help manage cholesterol levels.
- **Saturated Fats**: Found in red meat, butter, cheese, and many processed foods. These should be limited as they can raise bad cholesterol levels (LDL) and increase the risk of heart disease.
- **Trans Fats**: Found in many fried and commercially baked products. These are harmful fats that should be avoided as they significantly raise the risk of heart disease.

Incorporating Healthy Fats

Incorporating unsaturated fats into your diet can be as simple as using olive oil instead of butter, snacking on a handful of nuts, or adding avocado to your salads and sandwiches.

Portion Control

Even healthy fats are calorie-dense, so portion control is important. A small handful of nuts or a few slices of avocado is sufficient to gain the benefits without consuming excessive calories.

Micronutrients: The Small But Mighty Nutrients

Micronutrients, including vitamins and minerals, are required in smaller amounts but are vital for overall health. For diabetics over 50, certain micronutrients play a crucial role in managing the disease and promoting general well-being.

Key Vitamins and Their Sources

- **Vitamin D**: Essential for bone health and immune function. As we age, the skin's ability to synthesize vitamin D decreases. Sources include fortified dairy products, fatty fish, and sunlight exposure.
- **Vitamin B12**: Important for nerve function and the production of DNA and red blood cells. Found in animal products like meat, fish, dairy, and eggs. Older adults may need supplements due to decreased absorption.
- **Vitamin C**: Supports immune function and acts as an antioxidant. Found in citrus fruits, berries, bell peppers, and broccoli.
- **Vitamin E**: Acts as an antioxidant and helps with immune function. Found in nuts, seeds, and green leafy vegetables.

Essential Minerals and Their Sources

- **Calcium**: Crucial for bone health. Found in dairy products, fortified plant milks, and leafy greens.
- **Magnesium**: Supports muscle and nerve function and helps regulate blood sugar levels. Found in whole grains, nuts, seeds, and leafy green vegetables.
- **Potassium**: Helps maintain fluid and electrolyte balance and supports heart function. Found in bananas, potatoes, spinach, and beans.

- **Zinc**: Important for immune function and wound healing. Found in meat, shellfish, legumes, and seeds.

Antioxidants: Protecting Your Cells

Antioxidants help combat oxidative stress and inflammation, both of which are linked to diabetes and its complications. Foods rich in antioxidants include:

- **Berries**: Blueberries, strawberries, and raspberries.
- **Leafy Greens**: Spinach, kale, and Swiss chard.
- **Nuts and Seeds**: Almonds, walnuts, flaxseeds, and chia seeds.
- **Spices**: Turmeric, cinnamon, and ginger.

Hydration: The Often Overlooked Essential

Proper hydration is crucial for everyone, but especially for diabetics. Water is essential for maintaining blood volume, proper kidney function, and overall cellular health.

- **Water**: The best choice for staying hydrated without affecting blood sugar levels.
- **Herbal Teas**: Can be a flavorful alternative to water, but avoid those with added sugars.
- **Coffee and Tea**: Can be consumed in moderation, preferably without added sugars or high-fat creamers.

Tips for Balancing Macronutrients and Micronutrients

Balancing these nutrients involves thoughtful planning and mindful eating. Here are some practical tips:

1. **Create Balanced Plates**: Use the plate method where half of your plate is filled with non-starchy vegetables, a quarter with lean protein, and a quarter with whole grains or starchy vegetables.
2. **Snack Wisely**: Opt for snacks that combine protein and fiber, like an apple with almond butter or Greek yogurt with berries.
3. **Stay Informed**: Regularly read food labels to understand the nutritional content and avoid hidden sugars and unhealthy fats.
4. **Consult Professionals**: Work with a dietitian to tailor your diet to your specific needs, ensuring you get all necessary nutrients while managing blood sugar levels.
5. **Monitor Portions**: Use measuring tools or visual cues (like your hand) to keep portions in check.
6. **Variety Is Key**: Incorporate a wide range of foods to cover all nutrient bases and keep meals interesting.

Understanding macronutrients and micronutrients is fundamental for managing diabetes, particularly for those over 50. By focusing on complex carbohydrates, lean proteins, healthy fats, and essential vitamins and minerals, you can create a balanced diet that supports your health and helps control blood sugar levels. Remember, making informed food choices and maintaining a varied, balanced diet will not only improve your diabetes management but also enhance your overall quality of life.

GLYCEMIC INDEX EXPLAINED

The Glycemic Index measures how quickly and significantly a carbohydrate-containing food raises blood sugar levels after consumption. Foods are ranked on a scale from 0 to 100, with pure glucose assigned a reference value of 100. The index is divided into three categories:

- **Low GI (0-55)**: Foods in this range cause a slow, gradual rise in blood sugar levels.
- **Medium GI (56-69)**: These foods produce a moderate increase in blood sugar.
- **High GI (70-100)**: High GI foods lead to a rapid spike in blood sugar levels.

When we consume carbohydrates, they are broken down into glucose, the body's primary energy source. The rate at which this process occurs varies depending on the food's composition, fiber content, preparation method, and other factors. The Glycemic Index quantifies this rate by measuring the blood glucose response over two hours after eating a specific amount of carbohydrate (usually 50 grams).

Factors Influencing the Glycemic Index

Several factors can influence a food's Glycemic Index:

1. **Type of Carbohydrate**: Simple sugars like glucose and sucrose are quickly absorbed, resulting in a high GI. Complex carbohydrates, such as those found in whole grains and legumes, break down more slowly and have a lower GI.
2. **Fiber Content**: Foods high in dietary fiber, especially soluble fiber, tend to have a lower GI because fiber slows down the digestion and absorption of carbohydrates.
3. **Fat and Protein Content**: The presence of fats and proteins can slow carbohydrate digestion, leading to a lower GI.
4. **Processing and Preparation**: The more processed a food is, the higher its GI tends to be. For example, instant oats have a higher GI than steel-cut oats. Cooking methods also matter; al dente pasta has a lower GI than overcooked pasta.
5. **Ripeness**: The ripeness of fruits and vegetables can affect their GI. Ripe bananas have a higher GI than less ripe ones due to the higher sugar content as they ripen.

Glycemic Index vs. Glycemic Load

While the Glycemic Index is a useful tool, it does not take into account the amount of carbohydrates in a typical serving of food. This is where Glycemic Load (GL) comes into play. Glycemic Load considers both the quality (GI) and quantity of carbohydrates in a serving.

Foods with a low GL (10 or less) are considered to have a minimal impact on blood sugar levels, even if their GI is high. Conversely, foods with a high GL (20 or more) can significantly raise blood sugar levels.

Applications of the Glycemic Index

Incorporating the Glycemic Index into your daily diet can help manage blood sugar levels, especially for those with diabetes or prediabetes. Here are some practical tips:

1. **Choose Low-GI Foods**: Incorporate more low-GI foods into your diet. Examples include non-starchy vegetables, legumes, most fruits, whole grains, and dairy products.
2. **Combine Foods**: Pair high-GI foods with low-GI foods to balance the overall GI of your meal. For instance, add a side of lentils (low-GI) to a serving of rice (high-GI).
3. **Portion Control**: Be mindful of portion sizes. Even low-GI foods can cause a significant rise in blood sugar if consumed in large quantities.
4. **Opt for Whole and Minimally Processed Foods**: Choose whole grains over refined grains, fresh fruits over fruit juices, and minimally processed foods to maintain lower GI levels.
5. **Pay Attention to Preparation Methods**: Prefer cooking methods that preserve the integrity of carbohydrates, such as steaming or sautéing, rather than frying or mashing.

LOW, MEDIUM, AND HIGH GI FOODS

Low GI Foods (0-55)

- Lentils
- Chickpeas
- Non-starchy vegetables (broccoli, spinach, kale)
- Most fruits (apples, oranges, pears)
- Whole grains (barley, quinoa)
- Dairy products (milk, yogurt)
- Nuts and seeds

Medium GI Foods (56-69)

- Brown rice
- Whole wheat bread
- Sweet potatoes
- Pineapple
- Quick oats

High GI Foods (70-100)

- White bread
- White rice
- Russet potatoes
- Corn flakes
- Watermelon

Benefits of a Low-GI Diet

Adopting a low-GI diet offers numerous health benefits, particularly for individuals managing diabetes:

1. **Better Blood Sugar Control**: By choosing low-GI foods, you can prevent rapid spikes and drops in blood sugar levels, leading to better overall glycemic control.
2. **Improved Satiety**: Low-GI foods are digested more slowly, promoting a feeling of fullness and reducing the likelihood of overeating.
3. **Reduced Risk of Chronic Diseases**: A low-GI diet can help lower the risk of developing heart disease, stroke, and type 2 diabetes by improving blood lipid levels and reducing inflammation.

4. **Enhanced Weight Management**: The prolonged satiety associated with low-GI foods can support weight loss and maintenance, which is particularly important for managing diabetes.

Common Misconceptions

Misconception 1: Low GI Equals Low Carbohydrate

A common misconception is that low-GI foods are always low in carbohydrates. This is not necessarily true. For instance, lentils are low-GI but contain a significant amount of carbohydrates. The key is the rate at which these carbohydrates are absorbed.

Misconception 2: High GI Foods Should Be Completely Avoided

While it's beneficial to limit high-GI foods, they don't have to be eliminated. The overall balance and combination of foods in a meal are what matter most. For example, a high-GI food like watermelon can be paired with a low-GI food like yogurt to balance the meal's impact on blood sugar.

Misconception 3: All Sugars Are High GI

Not all sugars are high GI. Fructose, found in fruits, has a low GI. However, it's essential to consume sugars in moderation and focus on the overall nutritional profile of the food.

Glycemic Index

Incorporating the Glycemic Index into daily life involves making informed choices and planning meals that stabilize blood sugar levels. Here are some practical examples:

Breakfast
- **High GI**: Instant oatmeal with honey.
- **Low GI Alternative**: Steel-cut oats with fresh berries and a sprinkle of nuts.

Lunch
- **High GI**: White bread sandwich with processed meat.
- **Low GI Alternative**: Whole grain bread sandwich with lean turkey, avocado, and plenty of vegetables.

Dinner
- **High GI**: White rice with stir-fried vegetables.
- **Low GI Alternative**: Quinoa with grilled vegetables and a side of lentil salad.

Snacks
- **High GI**: Potato chips.
- **Low GI Alternative**: Carrot sticks with hummus.

This Glycemic Index is a useful tool for controlling blood sugar, especially for people over 50 who are just starting to make the dietary adjustments needed to manage their diabetes. One can enhance general health, lower the risk of complications from diabetes, and achieve improved blood sugar control by knowing how different meals affect blood glucose and making informed decisions. To fully reap the benefits of the Glycemic Index, balance your meals, include a variety of low-GI foods, and be mindful of portion sizes. Recall that the objective is to go closer to a better, more balanced diet that promotes your well-being rather than aiming for perfection.

PANTRY STAPLES FOR A DIABETIC DIET

Maintaining a well-stocked pantry is crucial for anyone aiming to manage diabetes through diet, especially for those over 50 who may have additional dietary needs. Having the right ingredients on hand can make meal preparation easier and ensure you have healthy options available at all times.

Whole Grains

- **Brown Rice**: Brown rice is a whole grain that retains its bran and germ, making it a more nutritious option than white rice. It has a lower glycemic index, which means it won't spike your blood sugar as rapidly. Use brown rice as a base for stir-fries, grain bowls, or as a side dish. It's versatile and can be cooked in large batches and stored for quick meals throughout the week.
- **Quinoa:** Quinoa is a protein-rich grain that's also high in fiber. It's gluten-free and has a low glycemic index, making it a great choice for diabetics. Quinoa can be used in salads, soups, or as a substitute for rice. It cooks quickly and has a pleasant, nutty flavor that complements a variety of dishes.
- **Steel-Cut Oats:** Steel-cut oats are less processed than rolled oats, which gives them a lower glycemic index. They make a hearty, satisfying breakfast that can help keep blood sugar levels stable. Top with berries, nuts, and a sprinkle of cinnamon for added flavor and nutrition. Oats can also be used in baking or to add texture to soups and stews.
- **Whole Wheat Pasta:** Whole wheat pasta is another excellent source of fiber and complex carbohydrates. It can be used in a variety of dishes from pasta salads to hearty main courses. Pair it with a protein source like chicken or tofu and plenty of vegetables to create a balanced, blood sugar-friendly meal.

Legumes

- **Lentils:** Lentils are packed with protein, fiber, and essential nutrients like iron and folate. They have a low glycemic index and can be used in soups, stews, salads, or as a meat substitute in dishes like shepherd's pie. Lentils cook relatively quickly and are available in several varieties, including green, brown, and red.
- **Chickpeas:** Chickpeas, or garbanzo beans, are incredibly versatile. They can be used in salads, soups, or made into hummus. Roasted chickpeas also make a great snack. High in protein and fiber, they help maintain stable blood sugar levels and keep you feeling full longer.
- **Black Beans:** Black beans are another nutritious legume, rich in protein and fiber. They're great in soups, stews, salads, and even as a base for veggie burgers. Like other legumes, they have a low glycemic index, making them ideal for blood sugar management.

Nuts and Seeds

- **Almonds:** Almonds are a great snack option for diabetics due to their high content of healthy fats, fiber, and protein. They can also be added to salads, yogurt, or oatmeal for extra crunch and nutrition. Be mindful of portion sizes, as nuts are calorie-dense.
- **Chia Seeds:** Chia seeds are tiny powerhouses of nutrition, offering a good amount of fiber, omega-3 fatty acids, and protein. They can be sprinkled on yogurt, added to smoothies, or used to make chia pudding. Chia seeds also help with blood sugar regulation by slowing the absorption of sugar in the bloodstream.
- **Flaxseeds:** Flaxseeds are rich in fiber and omega-3 fatty acids. They should be ground before consumption to ensure your body can absorb their nutrients. Add ground flaxseeds to smoothies, oatmeal, or baked goods. They also serve as an egg substitute in vegan baking.
- **Walnuts:** Walnuts are another excellent source of healthy fats, particularly omega-3 fatty acids. They can be eaten on their own, added to salads, or used in baking. Like other nuts, walnuts should be consumed in moderation due to their high-calorie content.

Healthy Oils and Fats

- **Olive Oil:** Olive oil is a staple of the Mediterranean diet, known for its heart-healthy monounsaturated fats. Use it for cooking, in salad dressings, or drizzled-over vegetables. Extra virgin olive oil is the least processed form and retains the most nutrients.
- **Avocado Oil:** Avocado oil is another healthy fat option, with a high smoke point that makes it suitable for cooking at high temperatures. It has a mild flavor that works well in salad dressings or as a cooking oil for stir-fries and roasted vegetables.
- **Coconut Oil:** Coconut oil contains medium-chain triglycerides (MCTs), which can provide quick energy. It's solid at room temperature, making it useful for baking and cooking. However, it should be used in moderation due to its high saturated fat content.

Spices and Herbs

- **Cinnamon:** Cinnamon has been shown to help lower blood sugar levels and improve insulin sensitivity. It can be added to oatmeal, smoothies, or baked goods. Incorporating cinnamon into your diet is an easy way to add flavor while potentially aiding blood sugar control.
- **Turmeric:** Turmeric contains curcumin, which has anti-inflammatory and antioxidant properties. It can be used in cooking a variety of dishes, from curries to soups. Pair it with black pepper to enhance the absorption of curcumin.
- **Garlic:** Garlic is known for its potential to improve heart health and lower blood sugar levels. It's a flavorful addition to many savory dishes, including stir-fries, soups, and roasted vegetables.
- **Ginger:** Ginger can help with digestion and has anti-inflammatory properties. It's great in teas, smoothies, and a variety of dishes. Fresh ginger adds a zesty kick, while ground ginger can be used in baking.

Sweeteners

- **Stevia:** Stevia is a natural sweetener derived from the leaves of the Stevia plant. It's calorie-free and doesn't raise blood sugar levels, making it a suitable sugar substitute for diabetics. Use it sparingly in beverages, desserts, and baking.
- **Monk Fruit:** Monk fruit sweetener is another natural, zero-calorie option that doesn't impact blood sugar levels. It can be used in the same way as stevia, offering a sweet taste without the negative effects of sugar.

Canned and Jarred Goods

- **Canned Tomatoes:** Canned tomatoes are a versatile pantry staple that can be used in sauces, soups, and stews. Look for low-sodium options to keep your salt intake in check. They provide vitamins and antioxidants, particularly lycopene.
- **Canned Tuna**: Canned tuna is a convenient source of lean protein. Opt for tuna packed in water rather than oil to reduce fat content. Use it in salads, sandwiches, or casseroles for a quick and nutritious meal.
- **Nut Butters:** Natural nut butter (like almond or peanut butter) without added sugars or hydrogenated oils is great for snacks and cooking. Spread on whole grain toast, add to smoothies, or use in baking. Be mindful of portion sizes due to their high-calorie content.

Baking Supplies

- **Whole Wheat Flour:** Whole wheat flour is a better alternative to white flour, as it retains more nutrients and fiber. Use it in baking breads, muffins, and other baked goods to increase their nutritional value.
- **Almond Flour:** Almond flour is low in carbs and high in healthy fats and fiber. It's perfect for gluten-free baking and adds a rich, nutty flavor to recipes. Use it in place of regular flour for a lower-carb option.
- **Coconut Flour:** Coconut flour is another low-carb, high-fiber alternative to traditional flour. It absorbs more liquid than other flours, so recipes need to be adjusted accordingly. It's great for making pancakes, muffins, and other baked goods.

Frozen Foods

- **Frozen Vegetables:** Having a variety of frozen vegetables on hand is a great way to ensure you always have healthy options available. They're just as nutritious as fresh vegetables and can be quickly steamed, roasted, or added to soups and stews.
- **Frozen Berries:** Frozen berries are perfect for adding to smoothies, oatmeal, or yogurt. They're packed with antioxidants and fiber, making them a great addition to a diabetic-friendly diet.
- **Frozen Fish Fillets:** Frozen fish fillets, such as salmon or cod, are convenient and nutritious options for quick meals. They're rich in omega-3 fatty acids and can be baked, grilled, or sautéed with your favorite seasonings.

MEAL PLANNING TIPS

The key to managing diabetes effectively is meal preparation, especially for those over 50 who are not accustomed to adjusting to new dietary restrictions. This procedure entails carefully weighing meal times, portion sizes, and dietary selections in order to support steady blood sugar levels all day. Learning how to prepare meals can greatly improve your health, regardless of your goals—regulating blood sugar, reaching a healthy weight, or just switching to a more balanced diet.

IMPORTANCE OF MEAL PLANNING
FOR DIABETICS OVER 50

Meal planning offers numerous benefits for individuals managing diabetes, especially those over 50 who may also be dealing with other age-related health concerns. Here are some key reasons why meal planning is crucial:

1. **Blood Sugar Control**: Planning meals in advance allows you to balance carbohydrates, proteins, and fats more effectively, which helps in regulating blood sugar levels. Consistency in meal timing and composition can prevent spikes and dips in blood glucose, promoting stable energy levels throughout the day.

2. **Portion Control**: As we age, our metabolism tends to slow down, making portion control even more critical. Meal planning encourages portion awareness, ensuring you don't overeat or consume excessive amounts of carbohydrates, which can lead to blood sugar fluctuations.

3. **Healthy Food Choices**: By planning your meals ahead of time, you can prioritize nutrient-dense foods such as vegetables, fruits, whole grains, lean proteins, and healthy fats. This approach minimizes reliance on processed foods high in sugars, unhealthy fats, and sodium, which are detrimental to overall health.

4. **Weight Management**: Maintaining a healthy weight is essential for managing diabetes effectively. Meal planning allows you to create balanced meals that support weight management goals without compromising on taste or satisfaction.

5. **Time and Convenience**: Planning meals in advance saves time during busy periods and reduces the temptation to opt for convenient but less healthy meal options. It also ensures you have the necessary ingredients on hand, minimizing last-minute grocery trips and stress.

Meal Planning Tips for Diabetics Over 50

1. **Set Realistic Goals**: Begin by setting achievable goals based on your individual needs, health status, and lifestyle. Whether your focus is on blood sugar control, weight loss, or overall health improvement, having clear objectives will guide your meal planning efforts.
2. **Understand Your Nutritional Needs:** Consult with a registered dietitian or healthcare provider to understand your specific nutritional requirements. Factors such as age, activity level, medications, and any other health conditions should be taken into account when planning meals.
3. **Use a Balanced Plate Approach:** Adopt the plate method as a visual guide for meal composition:

    - Fill half your plate with non-starchy vegetables like leafy greens, broccoli, and peppers.
    - Reserve a quarter for lean proteins such as chicken, fish, tofu, or legumes.
    - Allocate the remaining quarter for whole grains or starchy vegetables like brown rice, quinoa, or sweet potatoes.

4. **Choose Low-Glycemic Index Foods**: Opt for carbohydrates that have a lower glycemic index (GI), as they are digested more slowly and cause a gradual rise in blood sugar levels. Examples include whole grains (oats, barley), legumes (lentils, chickpeas), and most fruits (apples, berries).

5. **Include Lean Proteins:** Incorporate lean sources of protein into each meal to help stabilize blood sugar levels and promote satiety. Good options include poultry without skin, fish rich in omega-3 fatty acids (salmon, trout), tofu, and eggs.

6. **Emphasize Healthy Fats**: Include sources of healthy fats in your diet, such as avocados, nuts (almonds, walnuts), seeds (chia, flaxseed), and olive oil. These fats can improve cholesterol levels and reduce the risk of heart disease, common concerns for individuals with diabetes.

7. **Plan Meals around Vegetables**: Vegetables should be a central part of your meal planning. They are low in calories and carbohydrates, and high in fiber, vitamins, and minerals, making them an excellent choice for diabetes management. Experiment with different cooking methods and seasonings to enhance flavor without adding excessive salt or sugar.

8. **Prepare Ahead of Time**: Dedicate a specific time each week to plan your meals, create a shopping list, and prepare ingredients in advance. Consider batch-cooking larger portions of meals that can be stored and reheated throughout the week, saving time and ensuring you always have a healthy option on hand.

9. **Monitor Portion Sizes**: Use measuring cups, spoons, or a food scale to accurately portion out foods, especially carbohydrates. Overeating can lead to elevated blood sugar levels, so being mindful of portion sizes is crucial for managing diabetes effectively.

10. **Stay Hydrated:** Drink plenty of water throughout the day to stay hydrated. Avoid sugary beverages and limit caffeine intake, as these can affect blood sugar levels and hydration status.

11. **Read Food Labels**: Learn to read and interpret food labels to identify hidden sugars, unhealthy fats, and other ingredients that may impact your blood sugar control. Pay attention to serving sizes and the total carbohydrate content per serving.

12. **Be Flexible and Enjoy Variety:** Variety is key to maintaining a healthy diet. Experiment with different recipes, flavors, and cuisines to keep meals interesting and enjoyable. Incorporate seasonal produce and local ingredients to maximize freshness and nutritional value.

Meal planning that works with Individuals over 50 with diabetics, involves commitment, education, and a proactive attitude toward health maintenance. You may empower yourself to make well-informed dietary choices, accomplish optimal blood sugar control, and attain overall well-being by implementing these useful recommendations into your daily routine. Keep in mind that meal planning is an ongoing, dynamic process, so practice self-compassion.

<u>PORTION CONTROL</u>

Although portion control is crucial for controlling diabetes and maintaining general health, it's a notion that's frequently misinterpreted or ignored in our day-to-day eating routines. It involves more than just measuring food; it involves knowing how much to consume to support optimal health and maintain balanced blood sugar levels, particularly for those over 50 navigating the challenges of managing their diabetes.

Why Portion Control Matters
Portion control is crucial for several reasons, particularly for those with diabetes. Here's why:

- **Blood Sugar Management**: Controlling portion sizes helps regulate blood sugar levels throughout the day. Consuming large portions, especially carbohydrates, can lead to spikes in blood glucose, which is particularly risky for diabetics.

- **Weight Management**: Portion control aids in weight management or weight loss, which is often a goal for individuals with diabetes to improve insulin sensitivity and overall health.

- **Nutrient Balance**: By controlling portions, you ensure a balanced intake of macronutrients (carbohydrates, proteins, fats) and essential nutrients (vitamins, minerals) necessary for overall health.

- **Digestive Health**: Eating appropriate portions supports digestive health by preventing the overloading of the digestive system and promoting regularity.

Tips for Portion Control

Achieving portion control isn't about strict rules or deprivation; it's about making informed choices and developing mindful eating habits.

Here are practical tips to help you master portion control:

Use Portion Control Tools

- **Measuring Cups and Spoons**: Use these tools to measure grains, cereals, and liquids accurately.
- **Food Scale**: Weighing proteins and other foods can provide a clearer understanding of appropriate portion sizes.
- **Visual Comparisons**: Learn to estimate portion sizes using everyday objects (e.g., a deck of cards for meat servings, and a tennis ball for fruit).

Plate Method

The plate method is a visual guide to help you create balanced meals:

- **Half Plate Non-Starchy Vegetables**: Fill half your plate with colorful vegetables like leafy greens, broccoli, peppers, and tomatoes. These are low in calories and high in fiber and nutrients.
- **Quarter Plate Lean Protein**: Reserve a quarter of your plate for lean proteins such as chicken, fish, tofu, or beans. Protein helps you feel full and supports muscle health.
- **Quarter Plate Whole Grains or Starchy Vegetables**: The remaining quarter can include whole grains (brown rice, quinoa, whole wheat pasta) or starchy vegetables (sweet potatoes, corn, peas). These provide energy and fiber.

Mindful Eating Practices

- **Slow Down**: Eat slowly and savor each bite. This gives your body time to recognize when you're full, preventing overeating.
- **Pause between Bites**: Put down your utensils between bites and chew thoroughly. This allows you to enjoy your food and recognize satiety cues.
- **Listen to Hunger Cues**: Eat when you're hungry and stop when you're comfortably satisfied, not overly full.

Read Food Labels

- **Serving Sizes**: Pay attention to serving sizes on food labels. They often differ from what we might consider a typical portion.
- **Calorie and Nutrient Content**: Check the calories and nutrient content per serving to make informed choices about portion sizes.

Plan Ahead

- **Meal Planning**: Plan your meals and snacks ahead of time to ensure balanced portions and avoid impulsive eating.
- **Pre-portion Snacks**: Divide snacks into single servings in advance to prevent overeating straight from the package.

Be Mindful of Beverages

- **Caloric Drinks**: Beverages like soda, sweetened coffee drinks, and fruit juices can add significant calories and sugar without providing satiety. Opt for water, herbal tea, or unsweetened beverages.

Restaurant Strategies

- **Share Meals**: Split a dish with a dining companion or ask for a half portion when eating out.
- **Box Half**: Immediately box up half of your meal before you start eating to avoid the temptation to overeat.

PORTION CONTROL AND SPECIFIC FOOD GROUPS

Carbohydrates:
- Focus on Quality: Choose whole grains like oats, quinoa, and whole wheat over refined grains (white bread, white rice).
- Watch Portions: Measure or estimate portions of rice, pasta, and bread to manage carbohydrate intake.

Proteins:
- Lean Choices: Opt for lean cuts of meat, poultry without skin, fish, tofu, and legumes.
- Palm-Sized Portions: Aim for a portion of protein that is about the size and thickness of your palm.

Fats:
- Healthy Choices: Choose unsaturated fats like olive oil, avocado, nuts, and seeds.
- Limit Portions: While healthy, fats are calorie-dense, so watch portion sizes to avoid excess calories.

Vegetables:
- Load Up: Non-starchy vegetables are low in calories and high in fiber and nutrients, making them ideal for filling up your plate without overdoing it.

Gaining control over portion sizes is a journey that involves learning, practice, and self-awareness. You may effectively manage your diabetes, promote general health, and have a satisfying relationship with food by putting these strategies and tips into practice. Recall that portion control is about enabling yourself to make decisions that support and nurture your wellbeing rather than about limitation. You can develop enduring behaviors that support health and longevity with perseverance and patience.

READING FOOD LABELS

Anyone who manages their diet for health, especially those with diabetes, has to be able to read food labels. Comprehending the intricacies of ingredient lists, serving sizes, and hidden sugars or additives that may affect blood sugar levels and general health is just as important as comprehending the fundamentals of nutrition. With an emphasis on the most important information for diabetics, let's explore the art and science of reading food labels in detail.

The Basics of Food Labels

Food labels are designed to provide consumers with essential information about the product's nutritional content and ingredients. They are typically found on the packaging of all processed and packaged foods, including beverages. Understanding how to interpret these labels empowers individuals to make informed choices that align with their dietary needs and health goals.

Key Components of a Food Label:

- **Serving Size:** This indicates the recommended portion size of the food. All other nutritional information on the label is based on this serving size. It's essential to compare the serving size listed with the amount you consume to accurately assess your nutrient intake.
- **Calories:** The number of calories per serving gives you an idea of how much energy you'll get from consuming that portion of food. For diabetics, monitoring calorie intake is important for weight management and blood sugar control.
- **Nutrients**: Food labels list various nutrients and their amounts per serving. Key nutrients to focus on include:
- **Total Carbohydrates**: Diabetics need to pay attention to the total amount of carbohydrates, including sugars and dietary fiber. Fiber is beneficial as it slows down the absorption of sugars and can help manage blood sugar levels.

- **Sugars**: Look for both added sugars and natural sugars (like those in fruits and dairy). Diabetics should aim to limit added sugars as they can cause rapid spikes in blood glucose.
- **Proteins**: Important for maintaining muscle mass and overall health.
- **Fats**: Differentiate between saturated fats (which should be limited) and healthier unsaturated fats (which are beneficial in moderation).
- **Sodium**: Diabetics should monitor sodium intake, as high levels can contribute to hypertension and other health issues.
- **Ingredients List**: Ingredients are listed in descending order by weight. This means that the first ingredient listed is the most predominant by weight in the product. Pay attention to the types and quantities of sugars, fats, and additives present.

Deciphering the Ingredients List

While the nutrition facts panel gives you quantitative information about the food's contents, the ingredients list provides qualitative insights into what the product contains.

Here's what to look for:

1. **Sugar and Sweeteners**: Sugar can appear under various names such as sucrose, high-fructose corn syrup, glucose, fructose, and maltose. Diabetics should be cautious of products with sugars listed near the top of the ingredients list.
2. **Types of Fats**: Check for sources of unhealthy fats like saturated and trans fats, which should be limited. Look for healthier fats such as monounsaturated and polyunsaturated fats, typically found in oils like olive oil or sunflower oil.
3. **Additives and Preservatives**: Some additives, like artificial sweeteners or preservatives, may have minimal impact on blood sugar but can affect overall health. Ingredients like artificial colors or flavors might also be listed.
4. **Allergens**: Food labels must disclose common allergens such as nuts, dairy, soy, and wheat. Diabetics with allergies or sensitivities need to scrutinize these lists.

Tips for Effective Label Reading

- **Compare Similar Products**: When choosing between similar products, compare their nutritional labels to make the best choice for your dietary needs.

- **Look beyond Marketing Claims**: Labels boasting terms like "low-fat" or "sugar-free" can be misleading. Always verify the actual nutritional content to ensure it aligns with your health goals.

SMART SHOPPING TIPS

One of the most important things to do when starting a diet-based diabetes management program is to buy wisely when shopping for groceries. Your capacity to maintain stable blood sugar levels and support general health can be greatly impacted by the decisions you make at the grocery store. Below are helpful hints and techniques for confidently navigating the aisles and making decisions that complement your diabetes diet.

- **Plan Ahead**:Before heading to the grocery store, take some time to plan your meals for the week. Planning not only saves time but also helps you make healthier choices. Consider the following steps:

- **Create a Meal Plan**: Outline your breakfasts, lunches, dinners, and snacks for the week. This helps ensure you have all the necessary ingredients on hand.

- **Check Your Pantry**: Take inventory of what you already have and make a list of items you need to buy.

- **Consider Special Occasions**: Factor in any upcoming events or special dietary needs when planning your meals.

- **Make a Detailed Shopping List**: A well-organized shopping list is your best ally in the grocery store. Here's how to create an effective list:

- **Categorize Items**: Group items by sections of the store (e.g., produce, dairy, protein) to streamline your shopping trip.

- **Include Specific Quantities**: Note down the quantities needed for each item to prevent overbuying or running out too soon.

- **Prioritize Fresh Produce**: Plan to buy fresh fruits and vegetables that are in season for optimal flavor and nutrients.

- **Focus on Whole Foods**: When filling your shopping cart, prioritize whole foods that are minimally processed and nutrient-dense:

- **Fresh Produce**: Aim to fill half of your cart with a colorful variety of fruits and vegetables. Opt for leafy greens, berries, citrus fruits, and non-starchy vegetables like broccoli, spinach, and bell peppers.

- **Whole Grains**: Choose whole grains such as brown rice, quinoa, oats, and whole wheat bread over refined grains. These provide more fiber and nutrients.

- **Lean Proteins**: Select lean cuts of meat like skinless poultry, fish, and tofu. Legumes such as lentils and beans are excellent plant-based protein sources.

- **Healthy Fats**: Include sources of unsaturated fats like avocados, nuts (almonds, walnuts), seeds (chia, flaxseed), and olive oil.

- **Read Food Labels Carefully**: Understanding how to interpret food labels empowers you to make informed choices. Pay attention to:

- **Total Carbohydrates**: This includes sugars and fiber. Choose foods with a higher fiber content to help stabilize blood sugar levels.

- **Serving Size**: Be mindful of portion sizes, as they can affect your carbohydrate intake.

- **Added Sugars**: Limit foods with added sugars, syrups, or sweeteners, as they can cause blood sugar spikes.

- **Sodium Content**: Opt for low-sodium or no-added-salt options, especially in canned goods and packaged foods.

- **Choose Low-Glycemic Options**: Foods with a low glycemic index (GI) release glucose more slowly into the bloodstream, helping to maintain steady blood sugar levels. Look for:

- **Whole Fruits**: Berries, apples, pears, and citrus fruits generally have a lower GI compared to tropical fruits like pineapple and watermelon.

- **Vegetables**: Most non-starchy vegetables like leafy greens, broccoli, and cauliflower have a low GI.

- **Whole Grains**: Select whole grains like barley, quinoa, and whole wheat pasta over refined grains like white rice and white bread.

- **Navigate the Perimeter of the Store**: The perimeter of the grocery store typically houses fresh produce, meats, dairy, and whole foods. This is where you'll find the majority of diabetic-friendly options:

- **Produce Section**: Stock up on a variety of colorful fruits and vegetables.

- **Butcher Counter**: Choose lean cuts of meat and poultry.

- **Dairy Aisle**: Opt for low-fat or fat-free dairy products like yogurt and cheese.

- **Bakery**: Select whole grain breads and wraps.

- **Limit Processed and Sugary Foods**: Processed foods often contain added sugars, unhealthy fats, and higher sodium levels. To reduce your intake:

- **Check Ingredient Lists**: Avoid products with ingredients like high-fructose corn syrup, hydrogenated oils, and excessive salt.

- **Choose Healthy Snacks**: Instead of sugary snacks, opt for unsalted nuts, fresh fruit, or low-fat cheese for satisfying snacks between meals.

- **Avoid Sugary Beverages**: Opt for water, herbal teas, or unsweetened alternatives to soda and sugary juices.

- **Be Cautious with "Diabetic" or "Sugar-Free" Products**: While products labeled "diabetic" or "sugar-free" may seem like healthy choices, they can still contain artificial sweeteners or other additives that may affect blood sugar levels. Always read labels and consume these products in moderation.

- **Shop Mindfully**: Stick to your list avoid impulse purchases by sticking closely to your prepared list.

- **Shop When Not Hungry**: Shopping on an empty stomach can lead to less healthy choices.

Nutritional recommendations and product offerings may change over time. Stay informed about current research and dietary guidelines for diabetes management. Be open to trying new foods and recipes that fit within your dietary needs and preferences.

You can make your grocery shopping experience empowering and positive by implementing these wise shopping practices, which will help you manage your diabetes more effectively. Making wise decisions at the grocery shop establishes the groundwork for a healthy, well-balanced diabetic diet that promotes your general health and wellbeing.

Happy dining and shopping!

Chapter 1

BREAKFASTS

Breakfast is widely regarded as the most significant meal of the day because it determines our metabolism and energy levels. A healthy breakfast is essential for regulating blood sugar levels and promoting general health in those with diabetes. Diabetic persons can start their day with a healthy focus by consuming nutrient-dense, low-glycemic foods such fresh fruits and vegetables, lean meats, and whole grains. It is recommended that breakfast alternatives emphasize complex carbs, fiber, and healthy fats in order to give sustained energy and minimize blood sugar increases during the morning.

Classic Oatmeal with Berries

Serving: 1
Prep Time: 5 minutes
Cook Time: 10 minutes

Ingredients:
- 1/2 cup old-fashioned rolled oats
- 1 cup water or unsweetened almond milk
- Pinch of salt (optional)
- 1/2 teaspoon ground cinnamon
- 1/2 cup mixed berries (such as strawberries, blueberries, raspberries)
- 1 tablespoon chopped nuts (almonds, walnuts) or seeds (chia seeds, flaxseeds), optional
- 1 teaspoon honey or maple syrup (optional, for sweetness)

Preparation:
- Cook Oatmeal In a small saucepan, bring the water or almond milk to a boil.
- Stir in the rolled oats and a pinch of salt (if using).
- Reduce the heat to low and simmer, uncovered, stirring occasionally, for about 5-7 minutes or until the oats are tender and the mixture has thickened to your desired consistency.
- Add Cinnamon: Stir in the ground cinnamon during the last minute of cooking to infuse the oatmeal with flavor.
- Serve: Transfer the cooked oatmeal to a serving bowl.

- Top with mixed berries and chopped nuts or seeds, if desired.
- Drizzle with a teaspoon of honey or maple syrup for added sweetness, if desired.
- Serve warm and enjoy your nutritious and satisfying breakfast!

Nutritional Information:
- Calories: Approximately 250 kcal
- Carbohydrates: 45g
- Protein: 7g
- Fat: 5g
- Fiber: 8g
- Sugars: 8g
- Sodium: Varies depending on added salt

Notes:
This Classic Oatmeal with Berries recipe provides a balanced combination of complex carbohydrates, fiber, and antioxidants from the berries, which help in managing blood sugar levels and providing sustained energy throughout the morning. Adjust sweetness and toppings according to personal preference and dietary needs. Preparing this wholesome breakfast ensures a nutritious start to the day for diabetic individuals, focusing on managing blood sugar levels while enjoying delicious flavors and textures.

Greek Yogurt Parfait With Nuts And Seeds

Serving: 1
Prep Time: 5 minutes
Cook Time: 0 minutes

Ingredients:
- 1/2 cup Greek yogurt, plain, low-fat
- 1/4 cup mixed nuts (almonds, walnuts, pecans), chopped
- 1 tablespoon chia seeds
- 1 tablespoon ground flaxseeds
- 1/2 cup fresh berries (strawberries, blueberries, raspberries)
- 1 teaspoon honey (optional, for sweetness)
- Fresh mint leaves for garnish (optional)

Preparation:
- Prepare the Yogurt Base: In a bowl or parfait glass, spoon half of the Greek yogurt.
- Layer with Nuts and Seeds: Sprinkle half of the mixed nuts, chia seeds, and ground flaxseeds over the yogurt.
- Add Berries: Layer half of the fresh berries on top of the nuts and seeds.
- Repeat Layers: Repeat the layers with the remaining Greek yogurt, nuts, seeds, and berries.

Drizzle with Honey (optional):
- If desired, drizzle the top layer with honey for added sweetness.
- Garnish: Garnish with fresh mint leaves for a touch of freshness (optional).
- Enjoy immediately as a nutritious and delicious breakfast.

Nutritional Information:
- Calories: Approximately 350 kcal
- Carbohydrates: 25g
- Protein: 20g
- Fat: 20g
- Fiber: 10g
- Sugar: 15g

Tips:
Experiment with different types of nuts, seeds, or fruits based on your preferences or what you have'

Make Ahead: Prepare the parfait the night before and refrigerate in a sealed container to grab and go in the morning.

Dietary Considerations: This recipe is high in protein and fiber, making it a great option for a balanced breakfast for individuals managing diabetes. Adjust honey or skip it based on personal dietary needs.

This Greek Yogurt Parfait with Nuts and Seeds is not only satisfying and delicious but also packed with nutrients to start your day off right.

Veggie-Packed Breakfast Burrito

Serving: 2 burritos
Prep Time: 15 minutes
Cook Time: 15 minutes

Ingredients:
- 4 large eggs
- 1/4 cup diced bell peppers (any color)
- 1/4 cup diced onion
- 1/4 cup diced tomatoes
- 1/4 cup chopped spinach
- 1/4 cup shredded cheese (cheddar or mozzarella)
- Salt and pepper to taste
- 2 whole wheat tortillas (8-inch diameter)
- Cooking spray or olive oil for cooking

Preparation:
- Prepare Vegetables: Dice the bell peppers, onion, and tomatoes. Chop the spinach.
- Cook Vegetables: In a non-stick skillet over medium heat, spray with cooking spray or add a little olive oil. Add diced bell peppers and onions, and sauté for 3-4 minutes until softened.
- Add Spinach and Tomatoes: Add chopped spinach and diced tomatoes to the skillet. Cook for another 2 minutes until spinach is wilted and tomatoes are slightly softened.
- Scramble Eggs: In a bowl, whisk the eggs with salt and pepper. Push the vegetables to the side of the skillet and pour in the whisked eggs. Stir gently until the eggs are scrambled and cooked through, about 2-3 minutes.
- Assemble Burritos: Warm the whole wheat tortillas slightly in the microwave or on a dry skillet for 10-15 seconds to make them pliable. Divide the scrambled eggs and vegetable mixture evenly between the tortillas.
- Add Cheese: Sprinkle shredded cheese evenly over the eggs in each tortilla.
- Roll Burritos: Fold the sides of each tortilla toward the center, then roll it up tightly from the bottom to enclose the filling.
- Serve: Cut each burrito in half diagonally and serve warm.

Nutritional Information (per serving):
- Calories: 280 kcal
- Carbohydrates: 23g
- Fiber: 5g
- Sugars: 3g
- Protein: 18g
- Fat: 13g
- Saturated Fat: 5g
- Unsaturated Fats: 8g
- Cholesterol: 380mg
- Sodium: 450mg

Tips:
This Veggie-Packed Breakfast Burrito is not only delicious but also provides a good balance of protein, carbohydrates, and healthy fats, making it a nutritious choice for a diabetic-friendly breakfast. Customize the vegetables according to preference.

Avocado Toast on Whole Grain Bread

Serving: 2 slices of toast
Prep Time: 10 minutes
Cook Time: 5 minutes

Ingredients:
- 2 slices of whole grain bread
- 1 ripe avocado
- 1 tablespoon lemon juice
- Salt and pepper to taste
- Optional toppings: sliced cherry tomatoes, chopped cilantro, red pepper flakes

Preparation:
- Toast the Bread: Place the whole grain bread slices in a toaster or toaster oven. Toast until golden brown and crispy.
- Prepare the Avocado Spread: While the bread is toasting, halve the avocado and remove the pit. Scoop the avocado flesh into a small bowl.
- Add lemon juice, salt, and pepper to taste.
- Mash the avocado with a fork until smooth and creamy.
- Assemble the Avocado Toast: Once the bread is toasted, spread the mashed avocado evenly over each slice.
- If desired, sprinkle with optional toppings such as sliced cherry tomatoes, chopped cilantro, or a pinch of red pepper flakes for extra flavor and texture.
- Transfer the avocado toast to a plate and serve immediately while the bread is still warm and crispy.

Nutritional Information (per serving):
- Calories: Approximately 200 kcal
- Total Fat: 10g
- Saturated Fat: 1.5g
- Sodium: 200mg
- Total Carbohydrates: 24g
- Dietary Fiber: 8g
- Sugars: 2g
- Protein: 5g

Tips:
Choose whole grain bread with at least 3 grams of fiber per slice for added fiber content.
Avocado provides healthy monounsaturated fats that can help improve cholesterol levels.
Adjust seasoning and toppings according to personal taste preferences and dietary needs.
Enjoy this Avocado Toast on Whole Grain Bread as a satisfying and nutritious breakfast option that's suitable for managing blood sugar levels in individuals with diabetes.

Spinach and Feta Egg Muffins

Serving: Makes 12 muffins
Prep Time: 15 minutes
Cook Time: 20 minutes

Ingredients:

- 8 large eggs
- 1/2 cup milk (skim or low-fat)
- 1 cup fresh spinach, chopped
- 1/2 cup feta cheese, crumbled
- 1/4 cup red bell pepper, diced
- 1/4 cup onion, finely chopped
- Salt and pepper, to taste
- Cooking spray or olive oil for greasing muffin tin

Preparation:

- Preheat your oven to 350°F (175°C). Grease a 12-cup muffin tin with cooking spray or olive oil.
- Prepare Vegetables: In a skillet over medium heat, sauté the chopped spinach, red bell pepper, and onion until softened, about 3-4 minutes. Set aside to cool slightly.
- Whisk Eggs: In a large mixing bowl, whisk together the eggs and milk until well combined. Season with salt and pepper.
- Combine Ingredients: Stir in the cooked vegetables and crumbled feta cheese into the egg mixture until evenly distributed.
- Fill Muffin Tin: Pour the egg mixture evenly into the prepared muffin cups, filling each about 3/4 full.
- Bake: Place the muffin tin in the preheated oven and bake for 18-20 minutes, or until the egg muffins are set and lightly golden on top. They should puff up slightly and a toothpick inserted into the center should come out clean.
- Cool and Serve: Remove from the oven and allow the egg muffins to cool in the tin for a few minutes before carefully removing them. Serve warm.

Nutritional Information (per muffin):

- Calories: 78 kcal
- Total Fat: 5g
- Saturated Fat: 2g
- Cholesterol: 117mg
- Sodium: 125mg
- Total Carbohydrates: 2g
- Dietary Fiber: 0.3g
- Sugars: 1g
- Protein: 6g

Tips:

These spinach and feta egg muffins can be stored in an airtight container in the refrigerator for up to 3-4 days. They are perfect for meal prepping breakfasts for the week!

Feel free to customize with your favorite vegetables or herbs such as diced tomatoes, mushrooms, or fresh herbs like basil or parsley.

Cinnamon Quinoa Breakfast Bowl

Serving: 2 servings
Prep Time: 10 minutes
Cook Time: 15 minutes

Ingredients:
- 1/2 cup quinoa, rinsed
- 1 cup water
- 1/2 cup unsweetened almond milk (or any milk of your choice)
- 1/2 teaspoon ground cinnamon
- 1/4 teaspoon vanilla extract
- 1 tablespoon chopped walnuts
- 1 tablespoon chopped almonds
- 1 tablespoon ground flaxseed
- Fresh berries (such as strawberries, blueberries, or raspberries), for topping
- Optional: drizzle of honey or maple syrup (if desired)

Preparation:
- Cook Quinoa: In a small saucepan, bring the quinoa and water to a boil. Reduce heat to low, cover, and simmer for about 12-15 minutes, or until quinoa is tender and water is absorbed.
- Flavor with Cinnamon and Vanilla: Once quinoa is cooked, stir in the almond milk, ground cinnamon, and vanilla extract. Cook for an additional 2-3 minutes, stirring occasionally, until heated through and creamy.
- Assemble the Breakfast Bowl: Divide the cinnamon quinoa mixture between two bowls. Top each bowl with chopped walnuts, chopped almonds, ground flaxseed, and fresh berries.
- Optional Sweetener: If desired, drizzle a small amount of honey or maple syrup over each bowl for added sweetness.
- Serve: Enjoy your nutritious and delicious Cinnamon Quinoa Breakfast Bowl warm.

Nutritional Information (per serving):
- Calories: 250 kcal
- Carbohydrates: 30g
- Fiber: 5g
- Sugars: 3g
- Protein: 9g
- Fat: 11g
- Saturated Fat: 1g
- Monounsaturated Fat: 5g
- Polyunsaturated Fat: 4g
- Cholesterol: 0mg
- Sodium: 60mg
- Potassium: 320mg

Nutritional Benefits:
- Quinoa: A complete protein source, providing essential amino acids.
- Cinnamon: Helps regulate blood sugar levels and adds a warm, comforting flavor.
- Nuts and Seeds: Rich in healthy fats, fiber, and antioxidants.
- Berries: Packed with vitamins, minerals, and antioxidants, while being low in sugar.

This Cinnamon Quinoa Breakfast Bowl not only satisfies morning hunger but also supports stable blood sugar levels for individuals managing diabetes.

Chia Seed Pudding with Fresh Fruit

Serving: 2 servings
Prep Time: 5 minutes
Chill Time: 4 hours or overnight

Ingredients:
- 1/4 cup chia seeds
- 1 cup unsweetened almond milk (or any milk of choice)
- 1 tablespoon maple syrup or honey (optional, adjust to taste)
- 1/2 teaspoon vanilla extract
- Fresh fruits (such as berries, sliced banana, or mango) for topping
- Nuts or seeds (optional, for topping)

Preparation:
- Mix Chia Seeds and Liquid: In a bowl or jar, combine chia seeds, almond milk, maple syrup (if using), and vanilla extract. Stir well to combine, ensuring there are no clumps of chia seeds.
- Let it Sit: Cover the bowl or jar and refrigerate for at least 4 hours or overnight. During this time, the chia seeds will absorb the liquid and form a pudding-like consistency. Stir once or twice within the first hour to prevent clumping.
- Serve: When ready to serve, divide the chia seed pudding into two bowls or glasses.
- Add Toppings: Top each serving with fresh fruits of your choice. Berries, sliced banana, or mango are excellent options. Sprinkle with nuts or seeds for added texture and nutrition, if desired.
- Enjoy: Serve immediately and enjoy your nutritious and delicious chia seed pudding with fresh fruit!

Nutritional Information (per serving):
- Calories: Approximately 150 kcal
- Carbohydrates: 20g
- Fiber: 12g
- Sugars: 5g
- Protein: 5g
- Fat: 6g
- Saturated Fat: 0.5g
- Trans Fat: 0g
- Sodium: 80mg

Tips:
Adjust sweetness according to your preference by varying the amount of maple syrup or honey. Experiment with different toppings such as shredded coconut, cocoa nibs, or a drizzle of nut butter for variety.

Make a larger batch and store in the refrigerator for up to 3-4 days for quick breakfasts or snacks throughout the week.

This chia seed pudding with fresh fruit not only makes for a satisfying and nourishing breakfast but also provides a great source of fiber, healthy fats, and essential nutrients to support a diabetic-friendly diet. Enjoy the creamy texture and burst of flavors as you start your day on a healthy note!

Whole Wheat Pancakes with Blueberries

Serving: Makes about 6 pancakes
Prep Time: 10 minutes
Cook Time: 15 minutes

Ingredients:
- 1 cup whole wheat flour
- 1 tablespoon baking powder
- 1/4 teaspoon salt
- 1 tablespoon sugar substitute (optional)
- 1 cup low-fat milk or unsweetened almond milk
- 1 large egg
- 1 tablespoon melted butter or coconut oil
- 1 teaspoon vanilla extract
- 1/2 cup fresh blueberries (or frozen, thawed)

Preparation:
- Prepare the Batter:In a mixing bowl, whisk together the whole wheat flour, baking powder, salt, and sugar substitute (if using).
- In a separate bowl, beat the egg and then stir in the milk, melted butter or oil, and vanilla extract.
- Pour the wet ingredients into the dry ingredients and stir until just combined. Be careful not to overmix; it's okay if there are a few lumps.
- Gently fold in the blueberries.
- Cook the Pancakes:

- Heat a non-stick skillet or griddle over medium heat. Lightly grease with cooking spray or a little butter.
- Pour about 1/4 cup of batter onto the skillet for each pancake. Use the back of a spoon to spread the batter into a round shape.
- Cook for 2-3 minutes, or until bubbles form on the surface of the pancake and the edges look set.
- Flip the pancakes and cook for an additional 1-2 minutes, or until golden brown and cooked through.
- Transfer the pancakes to a plate and keep warm. Repeat with the remaining batter.
- Serve warm with a drizzle of sugar-free syrup, additional fresh blueberries, and a dollop of Greek yogurt if desired.

Nutritional Information (per serving):
- Calories: Approximately 150 kcal
- Carbohydrates: 25 g
- Fiber: 3 g
- Sugars: 3 g
- Protein: 6 g
- Fat: 4 g
- Saturated Fat: 2 g
- Cholesterol: 45 mg
- Sodium: 300 mg

Tips: Nutritional values are approximate and may vary depending on specific ingredients and portion sizes.

Smoked Salmon and Avocado Breakfast Plate

Serving:1
Prep Time: 10 minutes
Cook Time: 0 minutes (No cooking required)

Ingredients:
- 2 oz smoked salmon
- 1/2 ripe avocado, sliced
- 1 small tomato, sliced
- 1 hard-boiled egg, sliced
- 1/4 cup cucumber, sliced
- 1 tablespoon red onion, thinly sliced
- Fresh dill, for garnish
- Salt and pepper, to taste
- 1 teaspoon extra virgin olive oil
- 1 teaspoon lemon juice

Preparation:
- Slice the avocado, tomato, cucumber, hard-boiled egg, and red onion thinly. Set aside.
- If the smoked salmon is in large pieces, gently separate into bite-sized portions.
- Assemble the Breakfast Plate:
- Arrange the sliced avocado, tomato, cucumber, smoked salmon, hard-boiled egg, and red onion on a plate in a visually appealing manner.
- Drizzle the extra virgin olive oil and lemon juice over the avocado and vegetables.
- Season with salt and pepper to taste.
- Garnish with fresh dill for added flavor and presentation.
- Serve Immediately:

Nutritional Information (Per Serving):
- Calories: Approximately 300 kcal
- Protein: 20g
- Carbohydrates: 10g
- Fiber: 5g
- Sugar: 3g
- Fat: 20g
- Saturated Fat: 4g
- Cholesterol: 240mg
- Sodium: 450mg

Tips:
This breakfast plate is rich in protein and healthy fats from the smoked salmon and avocado, providing essential nutrients to start your day.
The combination of ingredients offers a balance of flavors and textures, perfect for those looking to manage blood sugar levels while enjoying a satisfying meal.
Feel free to customize the plate with your favorite herbs or additional vegetables to suit your taste preferences and nutritional needs.
This recipe not only caters to the nutritional requirements of diabetic patients but also ensures a flavorful and visually appealing breakfast option.

Mushroom and Spinach Omelet

Serving: Makes 1 omelet
Prep Time: 10 minutes
Cook Time: 10 minutes

Ingredients:

- 2 large eggs
- 1/4 cup sliced mushrooms
- 1/2 cup fresh spinach leaves
- 1 tablespoon chopped onion
- 1 teaspoon olive oil
- Salt and pepper to taste
- Optional: 1 tablespoon shredded cheese (low-fat or reduced-fat, if desired)

Preparation:

- Prepare Ingredients: Wash and slice the mushrooms, chop the onion, and rinse the spinach leaves thoroughly. If using cheese, grate or shred it and set aside.
- Cook Vegetables: Heat olive oil in a non-stick skillet over medium heat. Add chopped onion and sliced mushrooms. Sauté for about 3-4 minutes until mushrooms are tender and onions are translucent.
- Add Spinach: Add fresh spinach leaves to the skillet. Cook for another 1-2 minutes until spinach wilts. Season with salt and pepper to taste. Remove vegetables from skillet and set aside.
- Prepare Eggs: In a small bowl, whisk the eggs until well combined. Season with a pinch of salt and pepper.
- Cook Omelet: Wipe the skillet clean or use a separate skillet. Heat it over medium heat and add a drizzle of olive oil or cooking spray. Pour in the whisked eggs, swirling the pan to spread them evenly.
- Add Vegetables: Once the edges of the omelet begin to set, spoon the sautéed mushroom, spinach, and onion mixture evenly over one half of the omelet. Sprinkle with shredded cheese if using.
- Fold and Serve: Carefully fold the omelet in half with a spatula. Cook for another 1-2 minutes until eggs are fully cooked through and cheese (if added) is melted.

Nutritional Information (per serving):

- Calories: Approximately 220 kcal
- Carbohydrates: 4g
- Protein: 16g
- Fat: 15g
- Saturated Fat: 4g
- Fiber: 1g
- Sodium: 280mg

Tips:

For a heartier meal, serve the omelet with a side of whole grain toast or a small portion of fruit.

Chapter 2
SMOOTHIES & BEVERAGES

Smoothies and beverages are refreshing and nutritious options that can be enjoyed at any time of the day. They offer a convenient way to incorporate a variety of fruits, vegetables, and other wholesome ingredients into your diet. Smoothies are typically blended drinks made from a combination of ingredients such as fruits, vegetables, yogurt, milk or plant-based milk, and often include additional boosts like protein powder, seeds, or nuts. They are known for their smooth texture and versatility, allowing you to experiment with different flavors and nutrient combinations.

Beverages, on the other hand, include a wide range of drinks such as herbal teas, infused waters, freshly squeezed juices, and warm beverages like coffee and tea. These can be enjoyed for hydration, relaxation, or to complement a meal.

Both smoothies and beverages can be tailored to suit various dietary needs and preferences, making them a popular choice for those looking to maintain a balanced and nutritious diet. They provide an easy way to boost your intake of vitamins, minerals, fiber, and antioxidants, promoting overall health and well-being. Smoothies and beverages can also be customized to accommodate specific dietary requirements, such as low-sugar or dairy-free options, making them suitable for individuals with diverse nutritional needs.

Green Detox Smoothie

Serving: Makes 2 servings
Prep Time: 10 minutes
Cook Time: 0 minutes

Ingredients:
- 1 cup fresh spinach leaves
- 1/2 cup cucumber, peeled and chopped
- 1/2 cup celery, chopped
- 1/2 cup fresh parsley leaves
- 1/2 avocado, peeled and pitted
- 1 green apple, cored and chopped
- 1 tablespoon fresh ginger, peeled and grated
- Juice of 1/2 lemon
- 1 tablespoon chia seeds
- 1 1/2 cups unsweetened almond milk (or any preferred milk)

Preparation:
- Prepare the Ingredients: Wash the spinach, cucumber, celery, parsley, and apple thoroughly. Peel and chop the cucumber and celery. Core and chop the apple. Peel and grate the ginger. Pit and peel the avocado.
- Combine Ingredients: In a blender, add the spinach, cucumber, celery, parsley, avocado, apple, grated ginger, lemon juice, chia seeds, and almond milk.

- Blend Until Smooth: Blend on high speed until the mixture is smooth and well combined. If needed, add more almond milk to achieve desired consistency.

- Serve: Pour the green detox smoothie into glasses and serve immediately.

Nutritional Information (per serving):
- Calories: 120 kcal
- Carbohydrates: 15g
- Fiber: 7g
- Sugar: 6g
- Protein: 4g
- Fat: 7g

For added sweetness, you can include a small amount of honey or a few drops of liquid stevia, but be mindful of the total sugar content.

This smoothie is best consumed immediately after blending to retain its fresh flavor and nutrient content.

This green detox smoothie is not only delicious and refreshing but also packed with fiber, vitamins, and minerals that support overall health and are suitable for managing blood sugar levels in diabetic patients.

Berry Blast Smoothie

Serving: Makes 2 servings
Prep Time: 10 minutes
Cook Time: 0 minutes

Ingredients:
- 1 cup mixed berries (such as strawberries, blueberries, raspberries)
- 1/2 cup plain Greek yogurt (low-fat or non-fat)
- 1/2 cup unsweetened almond milk (or any preferred milk)
- 1 tablespoon chia seeds
- 1 tablespoon ground flaxseed
- 1 teaspoon honey or stevia (optional, for added sweetness)
- Ice cubes (optional, for desired consistency)

Preparation:
- Prepare the Ingredients: Wash the berries thoroughly under cold water. Remove any stems and hulls as necessary.
- Measure out the Greek yogurt, almond milk, chia seeds, and ground flaxseed.
- Combine Ingredients: In a blender, add the mixed berries, Greek yogurt, almond milk, chia seeds, and ground flaxseed.
- If using honey or stevia, add it to the blender for sweetness.
- Optionally, add a few ice cubes to achieve the desired thickness and chill.
- Blend Until Smooth: Secure the lid on the blender tightly.
- Start blending on low speed, gradually increasing to high speed until the mixture is smooth and creamy.
- Serve and Enjoy: Pour the Berry Blast Smoothie into glasses.
- Optionally, garnish with a few whole berries on top for presentation.
- Serve immediately and enjoy the refreshing and nutritious smoothie!

Nutritional Information (per serving):
- Calories: Approximately 120 kcal
- Carbohydrates: 15 grams
- Protein: 8 grams
- Fat: 4 grams
- Fiber: 6 grams
- Sugars: 8 grams
- Sodium: 70 mg

Tips: Nutritional values may vary depending on specific brands of ingredients and portion sizes.

This Berry Blast Smoothie is not only delicious but also packed with antioxidants, fiber, and protein, making it an excellent choice for a diabetic-friendly breakfast or snack. Enjoy the vibrant flavors and nutritional benefits while supporting stable blood sugar levels!

Protein-Packed Peanut Butter Smoothie

Serving: 1 serving
Prep Time: 5 minutes
Cook Time: 0 minutes

Ingredients:

- 1 ripe banana, frozen
- 1 tablespoon natural peanut butter (no added sugar or salt)
- 1 tablespoon flaxseeds or chia seeds
- 1 cup unsweetened almond milk (or any milk of your choice)
- 1/2 cup plain Greek yogurt
- 1/2 teaspoon vanilla extract (optional)
- Ice cubes (optional, for desired consistency)

Preparation:

- Prepare Your Ingredients: Gather all your ingredients and ensure your banana is frozen for a creamy texture.
- Blend Ingredients: In a blender, combine the frozen banana, natural peanut butter, flaxseeds or chia seeds, almond milk, Greek yogurt, and vanilla extract (if using).
- Blend Until Smooth: Blend on high speed until all ingredients are thoroughly combined and the smoothie reaches a creamy consistency. If desired, add ice cubes gradually and blend again until smooth.
- Serve: Pour the smoothie into a glass and enjoy immediately.

Nutritional Information:

- Calories: Approximately 350 kcal
- Protein: 20g
- Carbohydrates: 30g
- Fiber: 6g
- Sugar: 15g (from natural sources in banana and yogurt)
- Fat: 18g
- Saturated Fat: 3g
- Sodium: 180mg
- Potassium: 750mg

Tips:

Variations: You can customize this smoothie by adding a handful of spinach or kale for extra nutrients, or a scoop of protein powder for additional protein.

Adjust Consistency: If the smoothie is too thick, add more almond milk or water to achieve your desired consistency.

Diabetic-Friendly: This smoothie provides a good balance of carbohydrates, protein, and healthy fats, making it suitable for diabetic patients when consumed as part of a balanced meal plan.

Golden Turmeric Latte

Servings: 1
Prep Time: 5 minutes
Cook Time: 5 minutes

Ingredients:

- 1 cup unsweetened almond milk (or milk of choice)
- 1/2 teaspoon ground turmeric
- 1/4 teaspoon ground ginger
- 1/4 teaspoon ground cinnamon
- Pinch of black pepper (helps with turmeric absorption)
- 1 teaspoon honey or maple syrup (optional, adjust to taste)
- 1/2 teaspoon vanilla extract

Preparation:

- In a small saucepan, heat the almond milk over medium-low heat until warm but not boiling, stirring occasionally.
- Add the ground turmeric, ginger, cinnamon, black pepper, and vanilla extract to the warmed almond milk.
- Whisk the mixture gently until all the spices are well combined and the almond milk is heated through, about 2-3 minutes.
- Taste and adjust sweetness with honey or maple syrup if desired.
- Pour the Golden Turmeric Latte into a mug and sprinkle a dash of cinnamon on top for garnish.

Nutritional Information (per serving):

- Calories: 50 kcal
- Carbohydrates: 6g
- Fiber: 1g
- Sugars: 4g
- Fat: 2g
- Saturated Fat: 0g
- Protein: 1g
- Sodium: 180mg
- Potassium: 80mg

Tips:

Turmeric, ginger, and cinnamon are known for their anti-inflammatory properties and may help in managing blood sugar levels.

The addition of black pepper enhances the bioavailability of curcuming the active compound in turmeric.

Adjust sweetness levels to personal preference, keeping in mind the overall sugar content for diabetic dietary needs.

Enjoy this comforting and healthful Golden Turmeric Latte as a soothing beverage option that supports both taste and wellness goals for individuals managing diabetes.

Refreshing Cucumber and Mint Water

Serving: Makes about 4 servings
Prep Time: 10 minutes
Ingredients:

1 large cucumber, thinly sliced
1/4 cup fresh mint leaves
1 lemon, thinly sliced
4 cups cold water
Ice cubes (optional)

Preparation:
- Prepare the Ingredients: Wash the cucumber, mint leaves, and lemon thoroughly under cold water. Slice the cucumber and lemon into thin rounds.
- Combine Ingredients: In a large pitcher, add the sliced cucumber, mint leaves, and lemon slices.
- Add Water: Pour cold water into the pitcher over the ingredients.
- Infuse Flavors: Gently stir the mixture to combine. Let the ingredients infuse in the refrigerator for at least 1 hour, or preferably overnight, to allow the flavors to meld together.
- Serve: When ready to serve, fill glasses with ice cubes (if using) and pour the cucumber and mint water over the ice. Optionally, garnish each glass with a sprig of fresh mint or a slice of cucumber.

Nutritional Information (per serving):
- Calories: 0 (Water has negligible calories)
- Total Carbohydrates: 0g
- Fiber: 0g
- Sugars: 0g
- Protein: 0g
- Fat: 0g
- Sodium: 0mg

Tips:
Variations: Add a few slices of fresh ginger or a handful of berries for added flavor.
Storage: Keep refrigerated and consume within 2-3 days for best flavor.
Why This Recipe Works for Diabetic Patients:

Hydration: Cucumber and lemon provide refreshing hydration without added sugars or calories, helping to maintain stable blood sugar levels.
Low Glycemic Index: This drink is low in carbohydrates and has a low glycemic index, making it a suitable choice for diabetic patients.

Flavorful and Refreshing: The combination of cucumber and mint creates a refreshing drink that is enjoyable and helps encourage hydration throughout the day.

Enjoy this delightful and hydrating drink as part of a balanced diabetic diet, perfect for staying cool and refreshed while managing blood sugar levels effectively.

Spiced Chai Tea

Serving: 2 cups
Prep Time: 5 minutes
Cook Time: 10 minutes

Ingredients:
- 2 cups water
- 1 cinnamon stick
- 4 whole cloves
- 4 cardamom pods, lightly crushed
- 1-inch piece of fresh ginger, peeled and thinly sliced
- 2 black tea bags (regular or decaffeinated)
- 1 cup unsweetened almond milk (or any milk of your choice)
- 1-2 tablespoons honey or preferred sweetener (optional)
- Ground cinnamon, for garnish (optional)

Preparation:
- Boil Spices: In a small saucepan, bring the water to a boil. Add the cinnamon stick, cloves, cardamom pods, and sliced ginger. Reduce heat to low and simmer for 5 minutes to infuse the water with spices.
- Steep Tea: Remove the saucepan from heat and add the black tea bags. Let them steep for 3-5 minutes, depending on how strong you like your tea.
- Add Milk: Remove the tea bags and stir in the almond milk (or your choice of milk). If using honey or sweetener, stir it in until dissolved.
- Strain and Serve: Using a fine mesh sieve or tea strainer, strain the spiced chai tea into mugs or tea cups to remove the whole spices and ginger slices.
- Garnish and Enjoy: Optionally, sprinkle ground cinnamon on top for an extra hint of spice. Serve hot and enjoy your comforting spiced chai tea!

Nutritional Information (per serving):

- Calories: 30
- Total Fat: 1g
- Sodium: 60mg
- Total Carbohydrates: 5g
- Dietary Fiber: 1g
- Sugars: 3g
- Protein: 1g

Tips:
Adjust sweetness to your preference by adding more or less honey or sweetener.
You can store any leftover spiced chai tea in the refrigerator and reheat gently before serving.
This spiced chai tea recipe offers a warming and aromatic beverage option that's perfect.

Citrus Green Tea

Serving: 2 servings
Prep Time: 5 minutes
Cook Time: 5 minutes

Ingredients:
- 2 cups water
- 2 green tea bags
- 1/2 lemon, juiced
- 1/2 lime, juiced
- 1 tablespoon honey or agave syrup (optional, adjust to taste)
- Ice cubes
- Fresh mint leaves, for garnish (optional)

Preparation:
- Boil Water: In a small saucepan, bring 2 cups of water to a boil.
- Steep Green Tea: Remove the water from heat and add the green tea bags. Let them steep for 3-5 minutes, depending on desired strength.
- Cool Down: Remove the tea bags and allow the tea to cool to room temperature. You can speed up this process by placing the saucepan in the refrigerator for about 15 minutes.
- Prepare Citrus Juice: While the tea is cooling, juice half a lemon and half a lime into a small bowl or cup.
- Mix Ingredients: Once the tea has cooled, stir in the freshly squeezed lemon and lime juice. Add honey or agave syrup if desired, adjusting sweetness to taste.
- Serve: Fill two glasses with ice cubes. Pour the citrus green tea mixture over the ice cubes.
- Garnish: Optionally, garnish each glass with fresh mint leaves for a burst of freshness and aroma.

Nutritional Information (per serving):
- Calories: 10 kcal
- Carbohydrates: 3 g
- Sugars: 1 g
- Sodium: 5 mg
- Potassium: 20 mg

Tips: The nutritional information is approximate and may vary based on specific ingredients used and adjustments made to the recipe.

Enjoy this Citrus Green Tea as a refreshing and hydrating beverage that's not only delicious but also suitable for maintaining stable blood sugar levels. Adjust sweetness according to personal preference and health needs.

Almond Milk Smoothie with Chia Seeds

Serving: Makes 2 servings
Prep Time: 5 minutes
Cook Time: 0 minutes

Ingredients:
- 1 cup unsweetened almond milk
- 1 medium banana, frozen
- 1 tablespoon chia seeds
- 1 tablespoon natural almond butter
- 1 teaspoon pure vanilla extract
- 1/2 teaspoon ground cinnamon
- Ice cubes (optional, for desired consistency)

Preparation:

- Prepare Ingredients: Gather all your ingredients. If your banana is not frozen, you can add a few ice cubes to chill the smoothie.
- Combine Ingredients: In a blender, combine the unsweetened almond milk, frozen banana, chia seeds, almond butter, vanilla extract, and ground cinnamon.
- Blend Until Smooth: Blend on high speed until the mixture is smooth and creamy. If needed, add a few ice cubes to achieve your desired consistency.

- Serve: Pour the smoothie into glasses and garnish with a sprinkle of cinnamon or a few chia seeds if desired.

Nutritional Information (per serving):
- Calories: 150 kcal
- Carbohydrates: 20g
- Fiber: 6g
- Sugars: 8g
- Protein: 4g
- Fat: 7g
- Saturated Fat: 0.5g
- Trans Fat: 0g
- Sodium: 90mg
- Potassium: 320mg

Tips:

This smoothie is rich in fiber from the chia seeds and banana, providing sustained energy and aiding in digestion.

The almond milk and almond butter contribute healthy fats and a creamy texture without added sugars.

Enjoy this refreshing and nutritious Almond Milk Smoothie with Chia Seeds ial nutrients while keeping blood sugar levels stable.

Tomato and Basil Gazpacho

Serving: 4 servings
Prep Time: 15 minutes
Cook Time: 0 minutes (no cooking required)

Ingredients:

- 6 ripe tomatoes, chopped
- 1 cucumber, peeled, seeded, and chopped
- 1 red bell pepper, seeded and chopped
- 1 small red onion, chopped
- 2 cloves garlic, minced
- 2 cups tomato juice (low-sodium)
- 1/4 cup extra virgin olive oil
- 2 tablespoons red wine vinegar
- 1/4 cup fresh basil leaves, chopped
- Salt and pepper, to taste
- Optional garnish: diced cucumber, cherry tomatoes, basil leaves

Preparation:

- Prepare the Vegetables: In a large bowl, combine the chopped tomatoes, cucumber, red bell pepper, red onion, and minced garlic.
- Blend the Base: Transfer half of the vegetable mixture into a blender. Add half of the tomato juice, olive oil, red wine vinegar, and half of the chopped basil leaves. Blend until smooth.
- Combine Ingredients: Pour the blended mixture into a large serving bowl. Repeat with the remaining half of the vegetables, tomato juice, olive oil, vinegar, and basil. Blend until smooth and add to the serving bowl.
- Season to Taste: Stir the gazpacho well to combine. Season with salt and pepper to taste. Refrigerate for at least 1 hour to chill and allow the flavors to meld.
- Serve: Ladle the chilled gazpacho into bowls. Garnish with diced cucumber, cherry tomatoes, and additional basil leaves if desired. Serve cold and enjoy!

Nutritional Information (per serving):

- Calories: 180 kcal
- Total Fat: 14g
- Saturated Fat: 2g
- Trans Fat: 0g
- Cholesterol: 0mg
- Sodium: 310mg
- Total Carbohydrates: 15g
- Dietary Fiber: 3g
- Sugars: 9g
- Protein: 3g

Tips:

Enjoy this refreshing and nutritious Tomato and Basil Gazpacho as a light and satisfying meal or starter, perfect for warm weather or any time you crave a burst of fresh flavors!

Kale and Apple Juice

Serving: Makes about 2 servings
Prep Time: 10 minutes
Cook Time: 0 minutes

Ingredients:
- 2 cups kale leaves, tough stems removed
- 1 large apple, cored and chopped (choose a sweet variety like Fuji or Gala)
- 1 celery stalk, chopped
- 1 cucumber, peeled and
- 1/2 lemon, juiced
- 1-inch piece of chopped fresh ginger, peeled
- 1-2 cups water or coconut water (adjust for desired consistency)
- Ice cubes (optional)

Preparation:
- Prepare the Ingredients: Wash the kale leaves thoroughly and remove any tough stems. Chop the apple, celery, and cucumber into chunks.
- Juicing: In a high-speed blender, combine the kale leaves, chopped apple, celery, cucumber, fresh lemon juice, peeled ginger, and water (or coconut water).
- If using, add a handful of ice cubes for a chilled drink.
- Blend Until Smooth: Start blending on low speed and gradually increase to high speed until the mixture is smooth and well-combined. Blend for about 1-2 minutes, or until desired consistency is reached.
- Strain (Optional): If you prefer a smoother juice, strain the mixture through a fine mesh sieve or cheesecloth to remove any pulp.
- Pour the kale and apple juice into glasses and serve immediately. Optionally, garnish with a slice of lemon or a sprig of mint.

Nutritional Information (per serving):
- Calories: Approximately 80 kcal
- Total Fat: 0.5g
- Cholesterol: 0mg
- Sodium: 30mg
- Total Carbohydrates: 20g
- Dietary Fiber: 5g
- Sugars: 12g
- Protein: 2g

Tips:
This Kale and Apple Juice is rich in vitamins, minerals, and antioxidants, making it a refreshing and nutritious choice for diabetic patients.

Chapter 3
SALADS & DRESSINGS

Salads and dressings are versatile components of a healthy diet, offering a plethora of flavors, textures, and nutritional benefits. They are celebrated for their ability to incorporate fresh vegetables, fruits, proteins, and grains into a single dish, making them not only

Grilled Chicken and Avocado Salad

Serving: 4
Preparation Time: 15 minutes
Cook Time: 15 minutes

Ingredients
- 1 lb (450g) boneless, skinless chicken breasts
- 2 avocados, peeled, pitted, and sliced
- 4 cups mixed salad greens (such as spinach, arugula, and romaine)
- 1 cup cherry tomatoes, halved
- 1/2 cucumber, sliced
- 1/4 red onion, thinly sliced
- Juice of 1 lemon
- 2 tablespoons olive oil
- Salt and pepper, to taste
- Optional: fresh herbs (such as parsley or cilantro) for garnish

Preparation
- Preheat the Grill: Preheat your grill to medium-high heat.
- Grill the Chicken:
- Season the chicken breasts with salt and pepper.
- Grill the chicken for about 6-7 minutes per side, or until the internal temperature reaches 165°F (75°C) and the juices run clear.
- Remove from the grill and let it rest for 5 minutes before slicing it thinly.
- Prepare the Salad: In a large salad bowl, combine the mixed greens, cherry tomatoes, cucumber slices, and red onion.
- Add the sliced avocado to the salad bowl.
- Make the Dressing:In a small bowl, whisk together the lemon juice, olive oil, salt, and pepper.
- Assemble the Salad: Drizzle the dressing over the salad ingredients and gently toss to combine.
- Divide the salad evenly onto serving plates.
- Add Grilled Chicken: Arrange the sliced grilled chicken on top of each salad portion.
- Garnish and Serve: If desired, sprinkle with fresh herbs for garnish.
- Serve immediately and enjoy this nutritious and flavorful Grilled Chicken and Avocado Salad!

Nutritional Information (per serving)
- Calories: 320 kcal
- Carbohydrates: 14g
- Protein: 25g
- Fat: 19g
- Saturated Fat: 3g
- Cholesterol: 65mg
- Sodium: 280mg
- Fiber: 9g
- Sugar: 3g

Tips:
This not only satisfies the taste buds but also provides essential nutrients without compromising on health benefits. It's perfect for diabetic patients to stable blood sugar levels while enjoying a delicious and satisfying meal.

Quinoa and Black Bean Salad

Serving: 4 servings
Prep Time: 15 minutes
Cook Time: 20 minutes

Ingredients:
- 1 cup quinoa
- 2 cups water or low-sodium vegetable broth
- 1 can (15 ounces) black beans, drained and rinsed
- 1 cup cherry tomatoes, halved
- 1 bell pepper, diced (any color you prefer)
- 1/2 cup red onion, finely chopped
- 1/4 cup fresh cilantro, chopped
- Juice of 1 lime
- 2 tablespoons olive oil
- 1 teaspoon ground cumin
- Salt and pepper to taste
- Optional: avocado slices, for garnish

Preparation:
- Cook the Quinoa: Rinse the quinoa under cold water to remove any bitterness.
- In a medium saucepan, bring the water or vegetable broth to a boil.
- Add the quinoa, reduce heat to low, cover, and simmer for about 15 minutes, or until all liquid is absorbed and quinoa is fluffy. Remove from heat and let it cool.
- Prepare the Salad: In a large bowl, combine the cooked quinoa, black beans, cherry tomatoes, bell pepper, red onion, and cilantro.
- Make the Dressing: In a small bowl, whisk together the lime juice, olive oil, ground cumin, salt, and pepper.
- Combine and Toss: Pour the dressing over the quinoa and black bean mixture. Toss gently to combine and coat everything evenly with the dressing.
- Divide the salad into individual bowls or plates.
- Garnish with avocado slices if desired.

Nutritional Information (per serving):
- Calories: 320 kcal
- Total Fat: 9g
- Saturated Fat: 1g
- Cholesterol: 0mg
- Sodium: 250mg
- Total Carbohydrates: 50g
- Dietary Fiber: 10g
- Sugars: 2g
- Protein: 12g

Tips:
For added flavor, you can toast the quinoa in a dry skillet before cooking

Spinach and Strawberry Salad

Serving: 4
Prep Time: 15 minutes

Ingredients:

- 6 cups fresh spinach leaves, washed and dried
- 1 pint fresh strawberries, hulled and sliced
- 1/4 cup sliced almonds, toasted
- 1/4 cup crumbled feta cheese
- 2 tablespoons balsamic vinegar
- 1 tablespoon extra virgin olive oil
- 1 teaspoon honey (optional, adjust to taste)
- Salt and freshly ground black pepper, to taste

Preparation:

- Prepare the Ingredients: Wash and dry the spinach leaves thoroughly. Hull the strawberries and slice them. Toast the sliced almonds in a dry skillet over medium heat until lightly browned and fragrant.
- Make the Dressing: In a small bowl, whisk together the balsamic vinegar, extra virgin olive oil, honey (if using), salt, and pepper until well combined. Adjust seasoning to taste.
- Assemble the Salad: In a large salad bowl, combine the spinach leaves, sliced strawberries, toasted almonds, and crumbled feta cheese.

- Dress the Salad: Drizzle the prepared dressing over the salad ingredients. Gently toss the salad until everything is evenly coated with the dressing.
- Serve: Divide the salad among serving plates or bowls. Optionally, garnish with additional toasted almonds or feta cheese if desired.

Nutritional Information (per serving):

- Calories: 150 kcal
- Protein: 5g
- Carbohydrates: 12g
- Dietary Fiber: 4g
- Sugars: 6g
- Fat: 10g
- Saturated Fat: 2g
- Monounsaturated Fat: 6g
- Polyunsaturated Fat: 2g
- Cholesterol: 8mg
- Sodium: 200mg

Tips:

This Spinach and Strawberry Salad is not only delicious but also packed with nutrients. Spinach provides iron and vitamins, strawberries offer a dose of vitamin C and antioxidants, almonds add crunch and healthy fats, and feta cheese brings a creamy tanginess. Enjoy this refreshing and nutritious salad as a side dish or a light meal, perfect for supporting a balanced diabetic diet.

Mediterranean Chickpea Salad

Serving: 4
Prep Time: 15 minutes
Cook Time: 0 minutes

Ingredients:
- 2 cups cooked chickpeas (or 1 can, drained and rinsed)
- 1 cup cherry tomatoes, halved
- 1 cucumber, diced
- 1/2 red onion, thinly sliced
- 1/2 cup Kalamata olives, pitted and sliced
- 1/4 cup fresh parsley, chopped
- 1/4 cup fresh mint leaves, chopped
- 1/3 cup crumbled feta cheese (optional)

For the Dressing:
- 1/4 cup extra virgin olive oil
- 2 tablespoons red wine vinegar
- 1 clove garlic, minced
- 1 teaspoon dried oregano
- Salt and pepper to taste

Preparation:
- Prepare the Ingredients If using canned chickpeas, drain and rinse thoroughly under cold water.
- Halve the cherry tomatoes, dice the cucumber, thinly slice the red onion, chop the parsley and mint, and pit and slice the Kalamata olives.
- Make the Dressing: In a small bowl, whisk together the olive oil, red wine vinegar, minced garlic, dried oregano, salt, and pepper until well combined. Set aside.
- Assemble the Salad In a large mixing bowl, combine the chickpeas, cherry tomatoes, cucumber, red onion, Kalamata olives, chopped parsley, and chopped mint.
- Pour the dressing over the salad ingredients and gently toss until everything is evenly coated.
- Add Optional Feta Cheese: If using, sprinkle the crumbled feta cheese over the salad and toss gently to combine.
- Serve: Divide the Mediterranean Chickpea Salad into individual bowls or plates.
- Enjoy immediately as a refreshing and nutritious meal or side dish.

Nutritional Information (per serving):
- Calories: Approximately 280 kcal
- Protein: 9g
- Carbohydrates: 22g
- Fiber: 6g
- Sugar: 4g
- Fat: 18g
- Saturated Fat: 3g
- Monounsaturated Fat: 12g
- Polyunsaturated Fat: 2g
- Cholesterol: 8mg
- Sodium: 580mg

Kale Caesar Salad with Yogurt Dressing

Serving: 4 servings
Prep Time: 15 minutes
Cook Time: 0 minutes

Ingredients:
- 1 bunch of kale, washed and dried
- 1/4 cup plain Greek yogurt
- 2 tablespoons grated Parmesan cheese
- 1 tablespoon lemon juice
- 1 clove garlic, minced
- 1 teaspoon Dijon mustard
- Salt and pepper, to taste
- 2 tablespoons olive oil
- Optional: Croutons, cherry tomatoes, grilled chicken breast (for additional protein)

Preparation:
- Prepare the Kale: Remove the tough stems from the kale leaves and chop or tear the leaves into bite-sized pieces. Place them in a large salad bowl.
- Make the Dressing: In a small bowl, combine the Greek yogurt, Parmesan cheese, lemon juice, minced garlic, Dijon mustard, salt, and pepper. Mix well until smooth.
- Assemble the Salad: Pour the olive oil into the yogurt mixture while stirring continuously to emulsify the dressing.
- Pour the dressing over the kale leaves in the salad bowl. Use clean hands to massage the dressing into the kale leaves for about 1-2 minutes. This helps to tenderize the kale and evenly coat it with the dressing.
- Optional Additions: Add croutons, cherry tomatoes, or grilled chicken breast if desired, for added texture and flavor.
- Divide the salad into individual bowls or plates. Garnish with extra Parmesan cheese and freshly cracked black pepper if desired.

Nutritional Information (per serving):
- Calories: 120 kcal
- Protein: 6g
- Carbohydrates: 8g
- Fiber: 2g
- Sugars: 2g
- Fat: 8g
- Saturated Fat: 2g
- Cholesterol: 5mg
- Sodium: 160mg

Tips:
This is packed with nutrients like fiber, vitamins, and protein. It is without the excess calories and fat of traditional Caesar dressings.

Beet and Goat Cheese Salad

Serving: 4
Prep Time: 15 minutes
Cook Time: 1 hour (for roasting beets)

Ingredients:

- 4 medium beets, preferably golden or red
- 4 cups mixed salad greens (such as spinach, arugula, or spring mix)
- 1/2 cup crumbled goat cheese
- 1/4 cup chopped walnuts or pecans, toasted
- 1/4 cup balsamic vinegar
- 2 tablespoons extra virgin olive oil
- 1 tablespoon honey or maple syrup (optional, for dressing)
- Salt and pepper to taste

Preparation:

- Roast the Beets: Preheat the oven to 400°F (200°C).
- Scrub the beets clean under running water and pat dry with paper towels.
- Wrap each beet individually in aluminum foil and place on a baking sheet.
- Roast in the preheated oven for about 45-60 minutes, or until the beets are tender when pierced with a fork.
- Remove from the oven, unwrap the beets, and let them cool slightly. Once cool enough to handle, peel off the skins using your fingers (they should come off easily).
- Prepare the Dressing: In a small bowl, whisk together the balsamic vinegar, olive oil, honey or maple syrup (if using), salt, and pepper until well combined. Set aside.
- Assemble the Salad: Cut the roasted and peeled beets into wedges or slices.
- Arrange the mixed salad greens on a serving platter or individual plates.
- Top with the roasted beets, crumbled goat cheese, and toasted walnuts or pecans.
- Drizzle the prepared dressing over the salad just before serving.

Nutritional Information (per serving):

- Calories: 220 kcal
- Total Fat: 13g
- Saturated Fat: 4g
- Trans Fat: 0g
- Cholesterol: 10mg
- Sodium: 220mg
- Total Carbohydrates: 20g
- Dietary Fiber: 5g
- Sugars: 14g
- Protein: 8g

Tips:

Roasting Tips: Roasting the beets enhances their natural sweetness and brings out their earthy flavor. Be sure to wrap them individually in foil to prevent their juices from escaping.

Asian-Inspired Cabbage Slaw

Serving: 4 servings
Prep Time: 15 minutes
Cook Time: 0 minutes

Ingredients:
- 4 cups shredded cabbage (green or Napa cabbage)
- 1 cup shredded carrots
- 1/2 cup thinly sliced red bell pepper
- 1/4 cup chopped fresh cilantro
- 2 tablespoons toasted sesame seeds

For The Dressing:
- 2 tablespoons low-sodium soy sauce
- 1 tablespoon rice vinegar
- 1 tablespoon sesame oil
- 1 tablespoon fresh lime juice
- 1 teaspoon honey or maple syrup (optional)
- 1 teaspoon grated fresh ginger
- 1 clove garlic, minced
- Salt and pepper to taste

Preparation:
- Prepare the Vegetables: In a large mixing bowl, combine the shredded cabbage, shredded carrots, sliced red bell pepper, and chopped cilantro.
- Make the Dressing: In a small bowl, whisk together the soy sauce, rice vinegar, sesame oil, lime juice, honey (if using), grated ginger, minced garlic, salt, and pepper. Adjust seasoning to taste.
- Combine and Toss:Pour the dressing over the cabbage mixture in the large bowl. Toss well to coat evenly.
- Garnish: Sprinkle toasted sesame seeds over the slaw for added texture and flavor.
- Serve immediately as a refreshing side dish or chilled as part of a larger meal.

Nutritional Information (per serving):

- Calories: 80 kcal
- Total Fat: 4g
- Saturated Fat: 0.5g
- Trans Fat: 0g
- Cholesterol: 0mg
- Sodium: 350mg
- Total Carbohydrates: 9g
- Dietary Fiber: 3g
- Sugars: 4g
- Protein: 2g

Tips:
This Asian-Inspired Cabbage Slaw is not only vibrant in color but also packed with nutrients. The combination of cabbage, carrots, and bell peppers provides fiber and essential vitamins, while the sesame-ginger dressing adds a delightful tangy-sweet flavor.

For a complete meal, consider pairing this slaw with grilled chicken or tofu, or serve it alongside whole grain rice or noodles for added satiety.

Enjoy this refreshing and nutritious Asian-inspired slaw.

Cucumber And Dill Yogurt Salad

Serving: 4 servings
Prep Time: 15 minutes
Cook Time: 0 minutes

Ingredients:
- 2 large cucumbers, thinly sliced
- 1 cup plain Greek yogurt (low-fat or fat-free)
- 2 tablespoons fresh dill, chopped
- 1 tablespoon fresh lemon juice
- 1 clove garlic, minced
- Salt and pepper to taste

Preparation:
- Prepare the Cucumbers: Wash the cucumbers thoroughly under cold water. If desired, peel the cucumbers partially or completely, depending on personal preference.
- Slice the cucumbers thinly using a sharp knife or a mandoline slicer for uniform thickness.
- Make the Dressing: In a medium bowl, combine the Greek yogurt, chopped dill, fresh lemon juice, minced garlic, salt, and pepper. Stir well until all ingredients are thoroughly mixed.
- Combine Ingredients: Add the sliced cucumbers to the bowl with the yogurt dressing.
- Mix Thoroughly: Gently toss the cucumbers with the yogurt dressing until all slices are evenly coated.
- Chill (Optional):
- For enhanced flavor, cover the bowl with plastic wrap and refrigerate for at least 30 minutes before serving to allow the flavors to meld together.
- Serve the Cucumber and Dill Yogurt Salad chilled or at room temperature as a refreshing side dish or a light lunch option.

Nutritional Information (per serving):
- Calories: 70 kcal
- Total Fat: 1 g
- Saturated Fat: 0.5 g
- Cholesterol: 3 mg
- Sodium: 35 mg
- Total Carbohydrates: 8 g
- Dietary Fiber: 1 g
- Total Sugars: 5 g
- Protein: 8 g
- Vitamin D: 0 mcg
- Calcium: 100 mg
- Iron: 0.5 mg
- Potassium: 250 mg

Tips:
Adjust the amount of garlic and dill according to your taste preferences.

This salad can be made ahead and stored in the refrigerator for up to 2 days, though the cucumbers may release some water. Simply drain excess liquid before serving.

This Cucumber and Dill Yogurt Salad is not only low in calories and fat but also provides a good source of protein and essential nutrients, making it an excellent choice.

Roasted Vegetable Salad

Serving: 4 servings
Prep Time: 15 minutes
Cook Time: 30 minutes

Ingredients:

- 2 cups mixed vegetables (such as bell peppers, zucchini, red onion, and cherry tomatoes), chopped into bite-sized pieces
- 1 tablespoon olive oil
- Salt and pepper, to taste
- 4 cups mixed salad greens (lettuce, spinach, arugula)
- 1/4 cup crumbled feta cheese
- 2 tablespoons balsamic vinegar
- 1 tablespoon Dijon mustard
- 1 clove garlic, minced
- 1/4 cup extra virgin olive oil
- 1/4 teaspoon dried oregano
- 1/4 teaspoon dried basil
- Optional: 1/4 cup toasted walnuts or pine nuts

Preparation:

- Preheat the Oven: Preheat your oven to 400°F (200°C).
- Prepare Vegetables: Place the chopped mixed vegetables on a baking sheet. Drizzle with 1 tablespoon of olive oil and season with salt and pepper. Toss to coat evenly.
- Roast Vegetables: Roast in the preheated oven for about 25-30 minutes, or until the vegetables are tender and slightly caramelized, stirring halfway through cooking.
- Prepare Dressing: In a small bowl, whisk together balsamic vinegar, Dijon mustard, minced garlic, extra virgin olive oil, dried oregano, and dried basil until well combined.
- Assemble Salad: In a large bowl, combine the mixed salad greens with the roasted vegetables. Drizzle the dressing over the salad and toss gently to coat.
- Add Cheese and Nuts: Sprinkle crumbled feta cheese and toasted nuts (if using) over the salad.
- Serve: Divide the salad among plates and serve immediately.

Nutritional Information (per serving):

- Calories: 220 kcal
- Carbohydrates: 10g
- Fiber: 3g
- Sugar: 5g
- Protein: 4g
- Fat: 18g
- Saturated Fat: 4g
- Sodium: 240mg

Tips:

Vegetable Selection: Choose a colorful variety of vegetables for added nutrients and visual appeal.

Dressing Flavor: Adjust the amount of vinegar and mustard according to your taste..

Homemade Balsamic Vinaigrette

Serving: Makes about 1 cup of dressing
Prep Time: 5 minutes
Cook Time: 0 minutes

Ingredients:
- 1/2 cup extra virgin olive oil
- 1/4 cup balsamic vinegar
- 1 tablespoon Dijon mustard
- 1 clove garlic, minced
- 1 teaspoon honey or sugar substitute (optional, adjust to taste)
- Salt and freshly ground black pepper, to taste

Preparation:
- Combine Ingredients: In a small bowl or a glass jar with a lid, whisk together the olive oil, balsamic vinegar, Dijon mustard, minced garlic, and honey (if using). Alternatively, you can add all ingredients to a jar with a tight-fitting lid and shake vigorously until well combined.
- Season to Taste: Season with salt and freshly ground black pepper to taste. Adjust the sweetness with more honey or sugar substitute if desired.
- Store: Transfer the vinaigrette to a sealed container or jar. It can be stored in the refrigerator for up to 1 week.

Nutritional Information (per tablespoon):
- Calories: 80 kcal
- Total Fat: 9g
- Saturated Fat: 1g
- Trans Fat: 0g
- Cholesterol: 0mg
- Sodium: 20mg
- Total Carbohydrate: 1g
- Dietary Fiber: 0g
- Sugars: 1g
- Protein: 0g

Serving Suggestions:
- Drizzle over a fresh garden salad with mixed greens, tomatoes, cucumbers, and avocado.
- Use as a marinade for grilled vegetables or tofu.
- Toss with cooked quinoa or whole grain pasta for a flavorful side dish.

Tips:
Vary the Vinegar: Experiment with different types of vinegar such as red wine vinegar or apple cider vinegar for a unique twist.
Enhance with Herbs: Add chopped fresh herbs like basil, thyme, or parsley for added freshness and flavor.
Make Ahead: Prepare a larger batch and store in the refrigerator for quick and easy salad dressing throughout the week.
This homemade balsamic vinaigrette is not only delicious and versatile but also a healthy choice for those managing diabetes, ensuring you enjoy your meals without compromising on flavor or nutrition.

Chapter 4

SOUPS & STEWS

Soups and stews are beloved for their comforting warmth and versatility, making them perfect for any season. From hearty stews packed with wholesome ingredients to light, brothy soups bursting with flavors, these dishes offer a delicious way to enjoy nutritious meals. Whether you prefer a chunky vegetable stew or a silky smooth soup, soups and stews provide endless opportunities to showcase fresh ingredients while offering satisfying meals that are both wholesome and comforting.

Hearty Lentil Soup

Serving: Makes about 6 servings
Prep Time: 15 minutes
Cook Time: 40 minutes

Ingredients:

- 1 cup dried brown lentils, rinsed and picked over
- 1 tablespoon olive oil
- 1 medium onion, chopped
- 2 cloves garlic, minced
- 2 medium carrots, diced
- 2 celery stalks, diced
- 1 medium potato, peeled and diced
- 1 teaspoon ground cumin
- 1 teaspoon ground coriander
- 1/2 teaspoon smoked paprika
- 4 cups low-sodium vegetable or chicken broth
- 1 (14.5 oz) can diced tomatoes (no salt added)
- Salt and pepper to taste
- Fresh parsley or cilantro for garnish (optional)

Preparation:

- Cook Lentils: In a large pot, heat olive oil over medium heat. Add chopped onion and sauté until softened, about 5 minutes. Add minced garlic and cook for another minute until fragrant.
- Add Vegetables: Stir in diced carrots, celery, and potato. Cook for 5 minutes, stirring occasionally.
- Seasoning: Add ground cumin, coriander, and smoked paprika. Stir well to coat the vegetables with the spices.
- Simmer: Pour in the vegetable or chicken broth and diced tomatoes. Bring to a boil, then reduce heat to low. Cover and simmer for 30 minutes or until lentils and vegetables are tender.
- Season to Taste: Season with salt and pepper to taste. Adjust seasoning as needed.
- Serve: Ladle the soup into bowls. Garnish with fresh parsley or cilantro if desired.

Nutritional Information (per serving):

- Calories: Approximately 220 kcal
- Carbohydrates: 37g
- Fiber: 12g
- Sugars: 6g
- Protein: 12g
- Fat: 4g
- Saturated Fat: 0.5g
- Sodium: 300mg (if using low-sodium broth)
- Potassium: 800mg
- Vitamin A: 80% DV
- Vitamin C: 20% DV
- Iron: 15% DV

Tips:

Add Greens: Stir in a handful of chopped spinach or kale during the last few minutes of cooking for added nutrition.

Chicken And Vegetable Soup

Serving: 6 servings
Prep Time: 15 minutes
Cook Time: 30 minutes

Ingredients:
- 1 tablespoon olive oil
- 1 onion, finely chopped
- 2 cloves garlic, minced
- 2 carrots, diced
- 2 celery stalks, diced
- 1 red bell pepper, diced
- 1 zucchini, diced
- 1 teaspoon dried thyme
- 1 teaspoon dried oregano
- 1/2 teaspoon dried rosemary
- Salt and pepper to taste
- 6 cups low-sodium chicken broth
- 1 lb boneless, skinless chicken breasts, cut into bite-sized pieces
- 1 cup diced tomatoes (canned or fresh)
- 2 cups baby spinach leaves
- Fresh parsley, chopped, for garnish

Preparation:
- Heat olive oil in a large pot over medium heat. Add onion and garlic, sauté for 2-3 minutes until fragrant.
- Add carrots, celery, red bell pepper, and zucchini to the pot. Cook, stirring occasionally, for about 5 minutes until vegetables start to soften.
- Stir in dried thyme, dried oregano, dried rosemary, salt, and pepper. Cook for another minute until herbs are fragrant.
- Pour in chicken broth and bring to a boil. Add chicken pieces and diced tomatoes. Reduce heat to medium-low and simmer for 15-20 minutes until chicken is cooked through and vegetables are tender.
- Stir in baby spinach leaves and cook for 1-2 minutes until wilted. Taste and adjust seasoning if needed.
- Ladle the soup into bowls, garnish with fresh parsley, and serve hot.

Nutritional Information (per serving):
- Calories: 220 kcal
- Protein: 25g
- Carbohydrates: 12g
- Fiber: 3g
- Sugars: 5g
- Fat: 8g
- Saturated Fat: 1.5g
- Cholesterol: 60mg
- Sodium: 350mg

Tips: This Chicken and Vegetable Soup is a hearty and nutritious option for a diabetic-friendly meal. Packed with lean protein from chicken and a variety of colorful vegetables, it provides essential vitamins and minerals without excessive carbohydrates. The low-sodium chicken broth ensures a balanced flavor while keeping sodium intake in check..

Creamy Broccoli Soup

Serving: 4 servings
Prep Time: 15 minutes
Cook Time: 25 minutes

Ingredients:
- 1 tablespoon olive oil
- 1 medium onion, chopped
- 2 cloves garlic, minced
- 1 pound broccoli florets, chopped (about 4 cups)
- 1 medium potato, peeled and diced
- 3 cups low-sodium vegetable broth
- Salt and pepper, to taste
- 1/2 cup low-fat milk or unsweetened almond milk
- Optional toppings: Greek yogurt, chopped chives, grated low-fat cheese

Preparation:
- Sautéing Aromatics: In a large pot, heat olive oil over medium heat. Add chopped onion and sauté until translucent, about 3-4 minutes. Add minced garlic and sauté for another 1-2 minutes until fragrant.
- Adding Broccoli and Potato: Stir in chopped broccoli florets and diced potato. Sauté for 2-3 minutes, allowing flavors to meld together.
- Simmering: Pour in low-sodium vegetable broth. Bring the mixture to a boil, then reduce heat to low. Cover and simmer for 15-20 minutes, or until vegetables are tender.
- Blending: Use an immersion blender directly in the pot, or transfer the soup in batches to a blender. Blend until smooth and creamy.
- Seasoning: Season with salt and pepper to taste. Stir in low-fat milk or unsweetened almond milk to achieve desired creaminess.
- Serving: Ladle the soup into bowls. Optionally, garnish with a dollop of Greek yogurt, chopped chives, or grated low-fat cheese.

Nutritional Information (per serving):
- Calories: 150 kcal
- Total Fat: 5g
- Saturated Fat: 1g
- Trans Fat: 0g
- Cholesterol: 2mg
- Sodium: 320mg
- Total Carbohydrates: 23g
- Dietary Fiber: 5g
- Sugars: 4g
- Protein: 6g

Tips:
This Creamy Broccoli Soup is rich in fiber and vitamins, making it a nutritious choice for diabetic patients. The addition of potato helps provide a creamy texture without using heavy cream.

Tomato Basil Soup

Serving: 4 servings
Prep Time: 10 minutes
Cook Time: 30 minutes

Ingredients:
- 1 tablespoon olive oil
- 1 medium onion, chopped
- 2 cloves garlic, minced
- 2 cans (14.5 ounces each) diced tomatoes, preferably no-salt-added
- 1 can (6 ounces) tomato paste
- 2 cups low-sodium vegetable broth
- 1 teaspoon dried basil (or 1 tablespoon fresh basil, chopped)
- Salt and pepper to taste
- 1/2 cup low-fat milk or unsweetened almond milk (optional, for creaminess)

Preparation:
- Heat olive oil in a large pot over medium heat. Add chopped onion and cook until translucent, about 5 minutes.
- Add minced garlic and cook for another minute until fragrant.
- Stir in diced tomatoes (with their juices), tomato paste, vegetable broth, and dried basil. Bring to a simmer.
- Reduce heat to low and let the soup simmer for about 20-25 minutes, stirring occasionally, until flavors are well combined and soup has slightly thickened.
- If using, stir in low-fat milk or unsweetened almond milk for added creaminess. Season with salt and pepper to taste.
- Remove from heat and let the soup cool slightly.
- Using an immersion blender, blend the soup until smooth. Alternatively, carefully transfer the soup in batches to a blender and blend until smooth, then return to the pot.
- Serve hot, garnished with fresh basil leaves if desired. Enjoy!

Nutritional Information (per serving):
- Calories: 120 kcal
- Total Fat: 4g
- Saturated Fat: 0.5g
- Trans Fat: 0g
- Cholesterol: 0mg
- Sodium: 300mg
- Total Carbohydrate: 20g
- Dietary Fiber: 5g
- Sugars: 10g
- Protein: 3g

Tips:
This Tomato Basil Soup is rich in flavor yet low in calories and fat, making it a perfect choice for those managing diabetes or looking to enjoy a nutritious, comforting meal.

Minestrone Soup

Serving: 6
Prep Time: 15 minutes
Cook Time: 30 minutes

Ingredients

- 1 tablespoon olive oil
- 1 medium onion, diced
- 2 cloves garlic, minced
- 2 carrots, diced
- 2 celery stalks, diced
- 1 zucchini, diced
- 1 cup green beans, trimmed and cut into bite-sized pieces
- 1 can (15 ounces) diced tomatoes (preferably no salt added)
- 1 can (15 ounces) kidney beans, rinsed and drained
- 6 cups low-sodium vegetable broth
- 1 teaspoon dried oregano
- 1 teaspoon dried basil
- Salt and pepper to taste
- 1 cup small pasta (such as small shells or elbow macaroni)
- 2 cups fresh spinach, chopped
- Grated Parmesan cheese (optional, for garnish)

Preparation:

- Sauté Vegetables: In a large pot or Dutch oven, heat olive oil over medium heat. Add diced onion and cook until translucent, about 5 minutes. Add minced garlic and cook for another minute until fragrant.
- Add Vegetables: Stir in diced carrots, celery, zucchini, and green beans. Cook for about 5-7 minutes until vegetables begin to soften.
- Simmer Soup: Add diced tomatoes (with juices), kidney beans, vegetable broth, dried oregano, dried basil, salt, and pepper. Bring the soup to a boil, then reduce heat to low and simmer for 15-20 minutes, or until vegetables are tender.
- Cook Pasta: Meanwhile, cook the small pasta according to package instructions in a separate pot. Drain and set aside.
- Combine and Finish: Add cooked pasta and chopped spinach to the soup. Cook for an additional 2-3 minutes until spinach is wilted and pasta is heated through. Adjust seasoning with salt and pepper if needed.
- Serve: Ladle the minestrone soup into bowls. If desired, sprinkle with grated Parmesan cheese for added flavor (optional).

Nutritional Information (per serving)

- Calories: 250 kcal
- Carbohydrates: 45 g
- Fiber: 10 g
- Sugar: 7 g
- Protein: 10 g
- Fat: 5 g
- Saturated Fat: 1 g
- Trans Fat: 0 g
- Cholesterol: 0 mg
- Sodium: 400 mg

Spicy Black Bean Soup

Serving: 4 servings
Prep Time: 15 minutes
Cook Time: 30 minutes

Ingredients:
- 1 tablespoon olive oil
- 1 onion, finely chopped
- 2 cloves garlic, minced
- 1 jalapeño pepper, seeded and finely chopped (optional, adjust to taste)
- 1 red bell pepper, diced
- 2 teaspoons ground cumin
- 1 teaspoon chili powder
- 1/2 teaspoon smoked paprika
- 2 cans (15 ounces each) black beans, drained and rinsed
- 1 can (14.5 ounces) diced tomatoes, with juices
- 4 cups low-sodium vegetable broth
- Salt and pepper, to taste
- Fresh cilantro, chopped (for garnish)
- Greek yogurt or sour cream (optional, for serving)

Preparation:
- Sauté Aromatics: In a large pot, heat olive oil over medium heat. Add chopped onion and sauté until translucent, about 5 minutes. Add minced garlic and jalapeño (if using), and sauté for another 1-2 minutes until fragrant.
- Add Spices: Stir in ground cumin, chili powder, and smoked paprika. Cook for 1 minute, stirring constantly, until spices are toasted and fragrant.
- Combine Ingredients: Add diced red bell pepper, black beans, diced tomatoes (with juices), and vegetable broth to the pot. Stir well to combine.
- Simmer: Bring the soup to a boil, then reduce heat to low. Cover and simmer for 20-25 minutes, stirring occasionally, until flavors are well blended and vegetables are tender.
- Season to Taste: Season with salt and pepper to taste. Adjust seasoning and spiciness level as desired.
- Serve: Ladle the soup into bowls. Garnish with chopped fresh cilantro and a dollop of Greek yogurt or sour cream if desired.

Nutritional Information (per serving)
- Calories: 250 kcal
- Total Fat: 5g
- Saturated Fat: 1g
- Trans Fat: 0g
- Cholesterol: 0mg
- Sodium: 480mg
- Total Carbohydrates: 42g
- Dietary Fiber: 12g
- Sugars: 5g
- Protein: 13g

Turkey and Kale Stew

Serving: 4 servings
Prep Time: 15 minutes
Cook Time: 30 minutes

Ingredients:
- 1 lb ground turkey
- 1 tablespoon olive oil
- 1 onion, diced
- 2 cloves garlic, minced
- 2 carrots, peeled and diced
- 2 celery stalks, diced
- 1 teaspoon dried thyme
- 1 teaspoon dried rosemary
- 1/2 teaspoon smoked paprika
- Salt and pepper to taste
- 4 cups low-sodium chicken broth
- 1 can (14 oz) diced tomatoes, undrained
- 1 bunch kale, tough stems removed and leaves chopped (about 4 cups chopped)

Preparation:
- Brown Turkey: In a large pot or Dutch oven, heat olive oil over medium heat. Add ground turkey and cook until browned, breaking it up with a spoon as it cooks, about 5-7 minutes.
- Add Aromatics: Add diced onion, minced garlic, carrots, and celery to the pot. Cook, stirring occasionally, until vegetables are softened, about 5 minutes.
- Seasonings: Stir in dried thyme, dried rosemary, smoked paprika, salt, and pepper. Cook for 1 minute until fragrant.
- Simmer: Pour in chicken broth and diced tomatoes with their juices. Bring to a boil, then reduce heat to low and let simmer, uncovered, for 15 minutes.
- Add Kale: Add chopped kale to the pot. Stir well to combine. Simmer for an additional 5-7 minutes, or until kale is tender and wilted.
- Serve: Taste and adjust seasoning if needed. Ladle the stew into bowls and serve hot.

Nutritional Information (per serving):
- Calories: 280 kcal
- Carbohydrates: 14g
- Fiber: 4g
- Sugar: 5g
- Protein: 30g
- Fat: 12g
- Saturated Fat: 3g
- Trans Fat: 0g
- Cholesterol: 80mg
- Sodium: 560mg
- Potassium: 860mg

Tips:
Variation: Substitute ground turkey with lean ground chicken or beef, adjusting cooking time accordingly.
Storage: Store leftovers in an airtight container in the refrigerator for up to 3 days or freeze for longer storage.
Serve with: Enjoy this hearty stew on its own or with a side of whole grain bread for a complete meal.

Butternut Squash Soup

Serving: 6 servings
Prep Time: 15 minutes
Cook Time: 45 minutes

Ingredients:
- 1 medium butternut squash (about 2 lbs), peeled, seeded, and diced
- 1 onion, diced
- 2 cloves garlic, minced
- 1 medium carrot, diced
- 1 celery stalk, diced
- 4 cups low-sodium vegetable broth
- 1 teaspoon ground cinnamon
- 1/2 teaspoon ground nutmeg
- Salt and pepper, to taste
- 1 tablespoon olive oil
- Optional garnish: Greek yogurt and chopped fresh parsley

Preparation:
- Prepare the Squash: Start by peeling the butternut squash using a vegetable peeler. Cut it in half lengthwise, scoop out the seeds, and then dice the flesh into cubes.
- Sauté Vegetables: Heat olive oil in a large pot over medium heat. Add diced onion, garlic, carrot, and celery. Sauté for about 5-7 minutes until vegetables are softened and onions are translucent.
- Cook the Squash: Add the diced butternut squash to the pot. Season with cinnamon, nutmeg, salt, and pepper. Stir well to coat the vegetables with the spices.
- Simmer: Pour in the vegetable broth and bring the mixture to a boil. Reduce heat to low, cover, and simmer for about 30-35 minutes, or until the squash is tender and easily pierced with a fork.
- Blend: Remove the pot from heat and let it cool slightly. Using an immersion blender, blend the soup until smooth and creamy. Alternatively, transfer the soup in batches to a blender and blend until smooth (be cautious blending hot liquids).
- Adjust Consistency: If the soup is too thick, you can add a bit more vegetable broth or water to reach your desired consistency. Taste and adjust seasoning as needed.
- Serve: Ladle the hot soup into bowls. Garnish each serving with a dollop of Greek yogurt and a sprinkle of chopped fresh parsley, if desired.

Nutritional Information (per serving):
- Calories: 120 kcal
- Carbohydrates: 24 g
- Fiber: 4 g
- Sugars: 6 g
- Protein: 3 g
- Fat: 3 g
- Saturated Fat: 0.5 g
- Trans Fat: 0 g
- Cholesterol: 0 mg
- Sodium: 350 mg

Cabbage and Sausage Stew

Serving: 6 servings
Prep Time: 15 minutes
Cook Time: 30 minutes

Ingredients:

- 1 lb (450g) turkey sausage, sliced into rounds
- 1 tablespoon olive oil
- 1 onion, chopped
- 2 cloves garlic, minced
- 1 small head cabbage, cored and thinly sliced
- 2 carrots, peeled and sliced
- 1 can (14 oz / 400g) diced tomatoes
- 4 cups (1 liter) low-sodium chicken or vegetable broth
- 1 teaspoon dried thyme
- Salt and pepper to taste
- Fresh parsley, chopped (for garnish)

Preparation:

- Brown the Sausage: In a large pot or Dutch oven, heat olive oil over medium heat. Add the sliced turkey sausage and cook until browned, about 5-7 minutes. Remove sausage from the pot and set aside.
- Sauté Aromatics: In the same pot, add chopped onion and minced garlic. Sauté until onions are translucent and garlic is fragrant, about 3-4 minutes.
- Add Vegetables: Stir in sliced cabbage and carrots. Cook for another 5 minutes, stirring occasionally, until cabbage begins to wilt.
- Simmer: Pour in diced tomatoes (with their juices) and chicken or vegetable broth. Add dried thyme, salt, and pepper to taste. Bring the stew to a boil, then reduce heat to low. Cover and simmer for 15-20 minutes, or until vegetables are tender.
- Finish and Serve: Return the cooked sausage to the pot. Stir well to combine and heat through, about 2-3 minutes. Adjust seasoning if needed. Serve hot, garnished with chopped fresh parsley.

Nutritional Information (per serving):

- Calories: 250 kcal
- Protein: 15g
- Carbohydrates: 15g
- Fiber: 5g
- Sugars: 8g
- Fat: 15g
- Saturated Fat: 4g
- Trans Fat: 0g
- Cholesterol: 50mg
- Sodium: 650mg
- Potassium: 600mg

Tips:

Turkey Sausage: Opt for low-sodium or lean turkey sausage to reduce sodium and saturated fat content.

Mushroom Barley Soup

Serving: 6 servings
Prep Time: 15 minutes
Cook Time: 1 hour

Ingredients:
- 1 tablespoon olive oil
- 1 onion, diced
- 2 carrots, diced
- 2 celery stalks, diced
- 3 cloves garlic, minced
- 8 ounces mushrooms, sliced (any variety you prefer)
- 1 cup pearl barley, rinsed
- 8 cups low-sodium vegetable or chicken broth
- 1 teaspoon dried thyme
- 1 bay leaf
- Salt and pepper, to taste
- Fresh parsley, chopped (for garnish, optional)

Preparation:
- Sauté Vegetables: In a large pot or Dutch oven, heat olive oil over medium heat. Add diced onion, carrots, and celery. Sauté for 5-7 minutes until vegetables are softened and onions are translucent.
- Add Garlic and Mushrooms: Stir in minced garlic and sliced mushrooms. Cook for another 5 minutes, stirring occasionally, until mushrooms release their juices and begin to brown slightly.
- Add Barley and Broth: Add rinsed pearl barley to the pot. Pour in the low-sodium broth (vegetable or chicken, as per your preference). Stir in dried thyme and add the bay leaf. Season with salt and pepper to taste.
- Simmer: Bring the soup to a boil, then reduce the heat to low. Cover and simmer for 45-50 minutes, or until barley is tender and soup has thickened slightly. Stir occasionally to prevent sticking.
- Adjust Seasoning: Taste and adjust seasoning with salt and pepper if needed. Remove the bay leaf before serving.
- Serve: Ladle the mushroom barley soup into bowls. Garnish with fresh chopped parsley if desired. Serve hot and enjoy!

Nutritional Information (per serving):
- Calories: 220 kcal
- Total Fat: 4.5g
- Saturated Fat: 0.5g
- Trans Fat: 0g
- Cholesterol: 0mg
- Sodium: 350mg
- Total Carbohydrates: 40g
- Dietary Fiber: 8g
- Sugars: 5g
- Protein: 7

Chapter 5

MAIN DISHES

Main dishes are the centerpiece of a meal, typically comprising a protein source accompanied by complementary sides. These dishes often showcase diverse cooking techniques and flavor profiles, aiming to satisfy and nourish those enjoying them. Whether featuring meats, seafood, or plant-based proteins, main dishes offer a range of flavors and textures, making them an essential part of any dining experience.

Grilled Salmon with Lemon and Herbs

Serving: 4 servings
Prep Time: 15 minutes
Cook Time: 10 minutes

Ingredients:
- 4 salmon fillets, skin-on, about 6 ounces each
- 2 tablespoons olive oil
- 2 cloves garlic, minced
- 1 teaspoon lemon zest
- 2 tablespoons fresh lemon juice
- 1 tablespoon chopped fresh dill
- 1 tablespoon chopped fresh parsley
- Salt and pepper, to taste
- Lemon slices (for garnish)

Preparation:
- Preheat the Grill: Preheat your grill to medium-high heat. Make sure the grill grates are clean and lightly oiled to prevent sticking.
- Prepare the Marinade: In a small bowl, whisk together the olive oil, minced garlic, lemon zest, lemon juice, dill, parsley, salt, and pepper. This flavorful marinade will enhance the taste of the salmon.
- Marinate the Salmon: Place the salmon fillets in a shallow dish or a resealable plastic bag. Pour the marinade over the salmon, ensuring each fillet is evenly coated. Allow the salmon to marinate for about 10 minutes at room temperature. Marinating helps infuse the flavors into the fish.
- Grill the Salmon: Remove the salmon fillets from the marinade and place them skin-side down on the preheated grill. Discard any leftover marinade. Grill the salmon for about 4-5 minutes per side, or until the fish flakes easily with a fork and is cooked to your desired doneness. The skin should become crispy and golden brown.
- Serve: Transfer the grilled salmon to a serving platter or individual plates. Garnish with lemon slices for a fresh citrusy touch. Serve hot, alongside your favorite side dishes such as steamed vegetables, quinoa, or a leafy green salad.

Nutritional Information (per serving):
- Calories: Approximately 300 kcal
- Protein: 34g
- Fat: 17g (including healthy omega-3 fatty acids)
- Carbohydrates: 1g
- Fiber: 0.5g
- Sodium: 70mg

Tip: For those who prefer a lighter option, you can remove the salmon skin before grilling. This dish is not only delicious but also provides a healthy dose of protein and omega-3 fatty acids, which are beneficial for heart health and overall well-being.

Baked Chicken Breast with Vegetables

Serving: 4 servings
Prep Time: 15 minutes
Cook Time: 30 minutes

Ingredients:
- 4 boneless, skinless chicken breasts (about 1.5 lbs)
- 2 cups mixed vegetables (such as bell peppers, zucchini, and broccoli), chopped
- 2 tablespoons olive oil
- 2 cloves garlic, minced
- 1 teaspoon dried thyme
- 1 teaspoon dried rosemary
- Salt and pepper, to taste
- Fresh herbs (optional, for garnish)

Preparation:
- Preheat the oven to 400°F (200°C). Lightly grease a baking dish with olive oil or cooking spray.
- Prepare the Chicken: Pat the chicken breasts dry with paper towels and place them in the prepared baking dish.
- Drizzle 1 tablespoon of olive oil over the chicken breasts, then season both sides generously with salt, pepper, dried thyme, and dried rosemary.
- Rub the seasonings into the chicken breasts to ensure even coating.
- Prepare the Vegetables: In a large bowl, toss the chopped mixed vegetables with the remaining 1 tablespoon of olive oil, minced garlic, salt, and pepper.
- Spread the seasoned vegetables around the chicken breasts in the baking dish.
- Bake: Place the baking dish in the preheated oven and bake for 25-30 minutes, or until the chicken reaches an internal temperature of 165°F (75°C) and the vegetables are tender.
- Optional: For a golden-brown finish, broil the chicken and vegetables for an additional 2-3 minutes after baking.
- Remove from the oven and let it rest for a few minutes before serving.
- Garnish with fresh herbs if desired, such as chopped parsley or thyme.

Nutritional Information (per serving):
- Calories: 280 kcal
- Protein: 30g
- Carbohydrates: 8g
- Fiber: 3g
- Sugars: 3g
- Fat: 14g
- Saturated Fat: 2g
- Trans Fat: 0g
- Cholesterol: 80mg
- Sodium: 220mg

Tips:
Ensure chicken breasts are evenly sized for even cooking.
Feel free to vary the vegetables based on personal preference or seasonal availability.
Serve with a side of whole grains like quinoa or brown rice for a complete meal.
This Baked Chicken Breast with Vegetables recipe not only provides a delicious and satisfying meal but also aligns with a diabetic-friendly diet by focusing on lean protein and nutrient-rich vegetables.

Quinoa-Stuffed Bell Peppers

Serving: 4
Prep Time: 20 minutes
Cook Time: 40 minutes

Ingredients:

- 4 large bell peppers (any color)
- 1 cup quinoa, rinsed
- 1 ½ cups vegetable broth or water
- 1 tablespoon olive oil
- 1 onion, finely chopped
- 2 cloves garlic, minced
- 1 can (15 ounces) black beans, drained and rinsed
- 1 cup corn kernels (fresh or frozen)
- 1 teaspoon ground cumin
- 1 teaspoon chili powder
- Salt and pepper to taste
- 1 cup shredded cheese (optional, for topping)
- Fresh cilantro or parsley, chopped (for garnish)

Preparation:

- Preheat the Oven: Preheat your oven to 375°F (190°C).
- Prepare the Bell Peppers: Cut the tops off the bell peppers and remove the seeds and membranes.
- Place the peppers in a baking dish, standing upright.
- Cook Quinoa: In a saucepan, bring the vegetable broth or water to a boil.
- Add the quinoa, reduce heat to low, cover, and simmer for about 15 minutes or until quinoa is cooked and liquid is absorbed.
- Remove from heat and fluff with a fork.
- Prepare the Filling: In a large skillet, heat olive oil over medium heat.
- Add chopped onion and cook until softened, about 5 minutes.
- Add minced garlic, cumin, chili powder, salt, and pepper. Stir and cook for another minute until fragrant.
- Stir in black beans and corn kernels. Cook for 2-3 minutes until heated through.
- Combine Quinoa and Filling: Add the cooked quinoa to the skillet with the bean and corn mixture. Stir well to combine all ingredients evenly.
- Stuff the Peppers: Spoon the quinoa filling into each bell pepper, packing it down gently and filling to the top.
- If using cheese, sprinkle it over the stuffed peppers.
- Bake: Cover the baking dish with foil and place in the preheated oven.
- Bake for 30 minutes covered, then remove foil and bake for an additional 10 minutes or until peppers are tender and cheese (if using) is melted and bubbly.
- Remove stuffed bell peppers from the oven and let cool slightly.
- Garnish with chopped cilantro or parsley before serving.

Slow Cooker Beef Stew

Serving: 6 servings
Prep Time: 20 minutes
Cook Time: 6 hours on low or 3-4 hours on high

Ingredients:

- 1.5 lbs (680g) beef stew meat, cut into 1-inch cubes
- 2 tablespoons olive oil
- 4 cups low-sodium beef broth
- 1 cup red wine (optional; can substitute with additional beef broth)
- 1 onion, chopped
- 3 cloves garlic, minced
- 4 carrots, peeled and sliced
- 3 celery stalks, sliced
- 2 potatoes, peeled and diced
- 1 cup mushrooms, sliced
- 1 teaspoon dried thyme
- 1 teaspoon dried rosemary
- Salt and pepper, to taste
- 2 tablespoons cornstarch (optional, for thickening)
- Chopped fresh parsley, for garnish (optional)

Preparation:

- Brown the Beef: In a large skillet, heat 1 tablespoon of olive oil over medium-high heat. Add the cubed beef in batches, ensuring each piece is browned on all sides. Transfer the browned beef to the slow cooker.

- Prepare the Vegetables: In the same skillet, add the remaining tablespoon of olive oil. Sauté the onion and garlic until softened and fragrant, about 3-4 minutes. Transfer the onion and garlic mixture to the slow cooker.

- Combine Ingredients: Add the beef broth, red wine (if using), carrots, celery, potatoes, mushrooms, dried thyme, dried rosemary, salt, and pepper to the slow cooker. Stir gently to combine all ingredients.

- Cooking in the Slow Cooker: Low Setting: Cover and cook on low for 6 hours, or until the beef is tender and the vegetables are cooked through.

- High Setting: Alternatively, cook on high for 3-4 hours until the beef is tender.

- Thicken the Stew (Optional): In a small bowl, mix 2 tablespoons of cornstarch with 2 tablespoons of cold water until smooth. Stir the cornstarch mixture into the stew during the last 30 minutes of cooking to thicken the broth.

- Serve: Once cooked, taste and adjust seasoning with salt and pepper if needed. Serve the beef stew hot, garnished with chopped fresh parsley if desired.

Nutritional Information (per serving):

- Calories: 350 kcal
- Protein: 30g
- Carbohydrates: 25g
- Fiber: 4g
- Sugars: 5g
- Fat: 12g

Vegetable Stir-Fry with Tofu

Serving: 4 servings
Prep Time: 15 minutes
Cook Time: 15 minutes

Ingredients:

- 1 block (14 oz) firm tofu, drained and cut into cubes
- 2 tablespoons low-sodium soy sauce (or tamari for gluten-free option)
- 1 tablespoon rice vinegar
- 1 tablespoon cornstarch
- 2 tablespoons vegetable oil, divided
- 1 onion, thinly sliced
- 2 bell peppers (any color), thinly sliced
- 1 cup broccoli florets
- 1 cup snap peas, trimmed
- 2 cloves garlic, minced
- 1 tablespoon minced ginger
- Salt and pepper to taste
- Optional garnish: sesame seeds, sliced green onions

Preparation:

- Prepare Tofu: Start by pressing the tofu between paper towels or using a tofu press to remove excess moisture. Cut the tofu into cubes.
- Marinate Tofu: In a small bowl, mix together 1 tablespoon soy sauce, rice vinegar, and cornstarch. Toss the tofu cubes in this mixture until evenly coated. Set aside for 10 minutes to marinate.
- Cook Tofu: Heat 1 tablespoon of vegetable oil in a large skillet or wok over medium-high heat. Add the tofu cubes and cook until golden brown on all sides, about 5-7 minutes. Remove tofu from the skillet and set aside.
- Stir-Fry Vegetables: In the same skillet, heat the remaining tablespoon of vegetable oil. Add the sliced onion, bell peppers, broccoli florets, and snap peas. Stir-fry for 4-5 minutes until vegetables are tender-crisp.
- Flavoring: Add minced garlic and ginger to the skillet, stirring constantly for about 1 minute until fragrant.
- Combine: Return the cooked tofu to the skillet. Drizzle the remaining tablespoon of soy sauce over the mixture. Toss everything together gently until heated through and well combined.
- Seasoning: Season with salt and pepper to taste. Adjust seasoning if needed.
- Serve: Transfer the vegetable stir-fry with tofu to a serving dish. Garnish with sesame seeds and sliced green onions if desired.

Nutritional Information (per serving):

- Calories: 230 kcal
- Carbohydrates: 16g
- Fiber: 4g
- Sugar: 5g
- Protein: 15g
- Fat: 12g
- Saturated Fat: 1g
- Trans Fat: 0g

Turkey Meatballs with Zucchini Noodles

Serving: 4 servings
Prep Time: 20 minutes
Cook Time: 25 minutes

Ingredients:

- 1 pound ground turkey (preferably lean)
- 1/2 cup whole wheat breadcrumbs
- 1/4 cup grated Parmesan cheese
- 1 egg
- 2 cloves garlic, minced
- 1 teaspoon dried oregano
- 1/2 teaspoon dried basil
- Salt and pepper, to taste
- 2 tablespoons olive oil, divided
- 4 medium zucchinis, spiralized into noodles
- 2 cups marinara sauce (store-bought or homemade)
- Fresh basil leaves, chopped (for garnish)

Preparation:

- Preheat the oven to 400°F (200°C). Line a baking sheet with parchment paper or lightly grease it with olive oil.
- Make the Turkey Meatballs: In a large bowl, combine the ground turkey, breadcrumbs, Parmesan cheese, egg, minced garlic, dried oregano, dried basil, salt, and pepper. Use your hands to mix everything together until well combined.
- Roll the mixture into golf ball-sized meatballs (about 1.5 inches in diameter) and place them on the prepared baking sheet.
- Bake the meatballs in the preheated oven for 15-18 minutes, or until they are cooked through and lightly browned.
- Prepare the Zucchini Noodles: While the meatballs are baking, heat 1 tablespoon of olive oil in a large skillet over medium heat.
- Add the spiralized zucchini noodles to the skillet and sauté for 3-4 minutes, tossing frequently, until they are just tender. Season with a pinch of salt and pepper.
- Combine the Dish: Pour the marinara sauce into the skillet with the zucchini noodles and gently stir to coat the noodles evenly.
- Add the cooked turkey meatballs to the skillet with the zucchini noodles and marinara sauce. Heat everything together for another 2-3 minutes, until heated through.
- Serve: Divide the turkey meatballs and zucchini noodles among serving plates. Garnish with chopped fresh basil leaves.

Nutritional Information (per serving):

- Calories: 380 kcal
- Total Fat: 20g
- Saturated Fat: 5g
- Trans Fat: 0g
- Cholesterol: 120mg
- Sodium: 620mg

Baked Cod with Asparagus

Serving: 4 servings
Prep Time: 15 minutes
Cook Time: 20 minutes

Ingredients:
- 4 cod fillets (about 6 ounces each)
- 1 pound asparagus, trimmed
- 2 tablespoons olive oil
- 2 cloves garlic, minced
- 1 lemon (zested and juiced)
- 1 teaspoon dried thyme
- 1 teaspoon dried parsley
- Salt and pepper, to taste
- 1/4 cup grated Parmesan cheese (optional)
- Fresh parsley, chopped (for garnish)

Preparation:
- Preheat the Oven: Preheat your oven to 400°F (200°C). Line a baking sheet with parchment paper or lightly grease it with a bit of olive oil.
- Prepare the Asparagus: Place the trimmed asparagus on one side of the baking sheet. Drizzle with 1 tablespoon of olive oil and sprinkle with salt, pepper, and half of the minced garlic. Toss to coat evenly.
- Prepare the Cod Fillets: Pat the cod fillets dry with paper towels. Place them on the other side of the baking sheet, leaving some space between each fillet.
- Drizzle the cod fillets with the remaining 1 tablespoon of olive oil and sprinkle with salt, pepper, dried thyme, dried parsley, and the remaining minced garlic.
- Squeeze the juice of half a lemon over the cod fillets and asparagus. Sprinkle the lemon zest evenly over the top.
- Bake the Dish: Place the baking sheet in the preheated oven and bake for 15-20 minutes, or until the cod is opaque and flakes easily with a fork and the asparagus is tender.
- If using Parmesan cheese, sprinkle it over the asparagus and cod fillets during the last 5 minutes of baking to allow it to melt and become golden.
- Once baked, transfer the cod fillets and asparagus to serving plates. Garnish with fresh chopped parsley and serve with lemon wedges on the side for an extra burst of flavor.

Nutritional Information (per serving):
- Calories: 250 kcal
- Total Fat: 12g
- Saturated Fat: 2g
- Trans Fat: 0g
- Cholesterol: 60mg
- Sodium: 220mg
- Total Carbohydrates: 7g
- Dietary Fiber: 3g
- Sugars: 2g
- Protein: 30g

Tips:
Freshness: Choose fresh, firm cod fillets and bright green asparagus for the best results

Spaghetti Squash with Tomato Sauce

Serving: 4 servings
Prep Time: 15 minutes
Cook Time: 45 minutes

Ingredients:

- 1 large spaghetti squash
- 2 tablespoons olive oil, divided
- Salt and pepper, to taste
- 1 small onion, finely chopped
- 3 cloves garlic, minced
- 1 can (28 ounces) crushed tomatoes
- 1 teaspoon dried oregano
- 1 teaspoon dried basil
- 1/2 teaspoon dried thyme
- 1/4 teaspoon red pepper flakes (optional)
- Fresh basil leaves, chopped (for garnish)
- Freshly grated Parmesan cheese (optional)

Preparation:

- Preheat the Oven: Preheat your oven to 400°F (200°C). Line a baking sheet with parchment paper or lightly grease it with a bit of olive oil.
- Prepare the Spaghetti Squash: Carefully cut the spaghetti squash in half lengthwise and scoop out the seeds.
- Drizzle the cut sides of the squash with 1 tablespoon of olive oil and sprinkle with salt and pepper.
- Place the squash halves cut-side down on the prepared baking sheet.
- Bake in the preheated oven for 35-40 minutes, or until the squash is tender and easily pierced with a fork.
- Make the Tomato Sauce: While the squash is baking, heat the remaining 1 tablespoon of olive oil in a large skillet over medium heat.
- Add the chopped onion and sauté for 4-5 minutes, until softened.
- Add the minced garlic and cook for an additional 1-2 minutes, until fragrant.
- Pour in the crushed tomatoes and stir in the dried oregano, dried basil, dried thyme, and red pepper flakes (if using). Season with salt and pepper to taste.
- Bring the sauce to a simmer and let it cook for 15-20 minutes, stirring occasionally, until it thickens and the flavors meld together.
- Prepare the Spaghetti Squash Noodles: Once the squash is cooked, remove it from the oven and let it cool for a few minutes.
- Use a fork to scrape the flesh of the squash into long, noodle-like strands and transfer them to a large bowl.
- Combine and Serve: Add the tomato sauce to the bowl with the spaghetti squash noodles and toss gently to combine.
- Divide the spaghetti squash with tomato sauce among serving plates.
- Garnish with chopped fresh basil leaves and, if desired, a sprinkle of freshly grated Parmesan cheese.

Chicken and Broccoli Casserole

Serving: 4 servings
Prep Time: 20 minutes
Cook Time: 35 minutes

Ingredients:

- 2 cups cooked chicken breast, shredded or diced
- 4 cups broccoli florets
- 1 cup cooked quinoa
- 1 small onion, finely chopped
- 2 cloves garlic, minced
- 1 cup low-fat Greek yogurt
- 1/2 cup low-sodium chicken broth
- 1/2 cup shredded reduced-fat cheddar cheese
- 1/4 cup grated Parmesan cheese
- 1 teaspoon dried thyme
- 1 teaspoon dried parsley
- Salt and pepper, to taste
- 2 tablespoons olive oil, divided
- 1/4 cup whole wheat breadcrumbs (optional)

Preparation:

- Preheat the Oven: Preheat your oven to 375°F (190°C). Lightly grease a 9x13-inch baking dish with a bit of olive oil.
- Prepare the Broccoli: Bring a large pot of water to a boil. Add the broccoli florets and cook for 3-4 minutes until they are bright green and slightly tender. Drain and set aside.
- Sauté the Onions and Garlic: In a large skillet, heat 1 tablespoon of olive oil over medium heat. Add the finely chopped onion and sauté for 4-5 minutes until it becomes translucent.
- Add the minced garlic and cook for an additional 1-2 minutes until fragrant.
- Mix the Casserole: In a large bowl, combine the cooked chicken, blanched broccoli, cooked quinoa, sautéed onions and garlic, Greek yogurt, chicken broth, shredded cheddar cheese, grated Parmesan cheese, dried thyme, dried parsley, salt, and pepper. Stir until all ingredients are well incorporated.
- Assemble the Casserole: Transfer the mixture to the prepared baking dish, spreading it out evenly.
- In a small bowl, mix the whole wheat breadcrumbs with the remaining 1 tablespoon of olive oil. Sprinkle this mixture evenly over the top of the casserole for a crunchy topping (optional).
- Bake the Casserole: Place the baking dish in the preheated oven and bake for 25-30 minutes, or until the top is golden brown and the casserole is heated through.
- Remove the casserole from the oven and let it cool for a few minutes before serving. Garnish with fresh parsley if desired.

Nutritional Information (per serving):

- Calories: 320 kcal
- Total Fat: 12g
- Saturated Fat: 3g
- Trans Fat: 0g
- Cholesterol: 70mg
- Sodium: 380mg
- Total Carbohydrates: 25g

Shrimp and Avocado Tacos

Serving: 4 servings
Prep Time: 20 minutes
Cook Time: 10 minutes

Ingredients:

- 1 pound large shrimp, peeled and deveined
- 1 tablespoon olive oil
- 1 teaspoon chili powder
- 1/2 teaspoon cumin
- 1/2 teaspoon smoked paprika
- 1/4 teaspoon garlic powder
- Salt and pepper, to taste
- 8 small whole wheat or corn tortillas
- 2 ripe avocados, sliced
- 1 cup shredded red cabbage
- 1/2 cup chopped fresh cilantro
- 1/4 cup finely diced red onion
- 1 lime, cut into wedges
- 1/2 cup low-fat Greek yogurt
- 1 tablespoon lime juice
- 1 teaspoon hot sauce (optional)

Preparation:

- Prepare the Shrimp: In a medium bowl, combine the shrimp, olive oil, chili powder, cumin, smoked paprika, garlic powder, salt, and pepper. Toss until the shrimp are evenly coated with the spices.
- Cook the Shrimp: Heat a large skillet over medium-high heat. Add the shrimp to the skillet in a single layer.
- Cook for 2-3 minutes on each side, or until the shrimp are opaque and cooked through. Remove from heat and set aside.
- Prepare the Avocado: Slice the avocados in half, remove the pits, and slice the flesh into thin strips.
- Make the Lime Yogurt Sauce: In a small bowl, whisk together the Greek yogurt, lime juice, and hot sauce (if using) until smooth. Set aside.
- Warm the Tortillas: Warm the tortillas in a dry skillet over medium heat for about 30 seconds on each side, or until they are pliable and slightly browned. Alternatively, you can wrap them in a damp paper towel and microwave for 20-30 seconds.
- Assemble the Tacos: Place a few shrimp in the center of each tortilla.
- Top with sliced avocado, shredded red cabbage, chopped cilantro, and diced red onion.
- Drizzle with the lime yogurt sauce.
- Serve the tacos immediately with lime wedges on the side for squeezing over the top.

Nutritional Information (per serving):

- alories: 320 kcal
- Total Fat: 17g
- Saturated Fat: 3g
- Trans Fat: 0g
- Cholesterol: 170mg
- Sodium: 450mg
- Total Carbohydrates: 24g
- Dietary Fiber: 8g
- Sugars:

CHAPTER 6

SIDE DISHES

Side Dishes Introduction

Side dishes play a crucial role in enhancing any meal, providing balance and variety in flavors, textures, and nutritional content. For diabetic patients, choosing the right side dishes is essential to maintain blood sugar levels while ensuring a well-rounded diet.

In this section, you'll find an array of delicious and healthy side dishes that complement main courses beautifully. These recipes are designed with careful consideration of their glycemic impact, incorporating plenty of vegetables, whole grains, and lean proteins. Whether you're looking to add a crunchy salad, a savory vegetable medley, or a wholesome grain dish, these side dishes will enrich your meals with nutrients and delightful tastes, making every dining experience satisfying and health-conscious.

Garlic Roasted Brussels Sprouts

Serving: 4 servings
Prep Time: 10 minutes
Cook Time: 25 minutes

Ingredients:

- 1 pound Brussels sprouts, trimmed and halved
- 3 tablespoons olive oil
- 4 cloves garlic, minced
- Salt and pepper, to taste
- 1/4 teaspoon red pepper flakes (optional)
- 1 tablespoon balsamic vinegar
- Freshly grated Parmesan cheese (optional)
- Fresh parsley, chopped (for garnish)

Preparation:

- Preheat the Oven:Preheat your oven to 400°F (200°C). Line a baking sheet with parchment paper or lightly grease it with olive oil.
- Prepare the Brussels Sprouts: Place the halved Brussels sprouts in a large bowl. Add the olive oil, minced garlic, salt, pepper, and red pepper flakes (if using). Toss to coat the Brussels sprouts evenly with the oil and seasonings.
- Roast the Brussels Sprouts: Spread the Brussels sprouts in a single layer on the prepared baking sheet. Make sure they are not too crowded to ensure even roasting.
- Roast in the preheated oven for 20-25 minutes, stirring halfway through, until the Brussels sprouts are golden brown and crispy on the edges.
- Finish with Balsamic Vinegar: Remove the Brussels sprouts from the oven and immediately drizzle with balsamic vinegar. Toss to coat evenly.
- Transfer the roasted Brussels sprouts to a serving dish. If desired, sprinkle with freshly grated Parmesan cheese and garnish with chopped fresh parsley.

Nutritional Information (per serving):

- Calories: 150 kcal
- Total Fat: 10g
- Saturated Fat: 1.5g
- Trans Fat: 0g
- Cholesterol: 0mg
- Sodium: 50mg
- Total Carbohydrates: 12g
- Dietary Fiber: 4g
- Sugars: 2g
- Protein: 3g

Tips:

Even Roasting: Ensure Brussels sprouts are evenly coated with oil and not too crowded on the baking sheet to promote even roasting and prevent steaming.

Flavor Boost: For an extra flavor boost, add a squeeze of fresh lemon juice before serving.

Cauliflower Rice Pilaf

Serving: 4 servings
Prep Time: 15 minutes
Cook Time: 15 minutes

Ingredients:
- 1 large head of cauliflower
- 2 tablespoons olive oil
- 1 small onion, finely chopped
- 2 cloves garlic, minced
- 1 carrot, finely diced
- 1 celery stalk, finely diced
- 1/2 cup frozen peas, thawed
- 1/4 cup slivered almonds, toasted
- 1/4 cup chopped fresh parsley
- 1 teaspoon dried thyme
- 1/2 teaspoon dried oregano
- Salt and pepper, to taste
- Juice of 1 lemon

Preparation:
- Prepare the Cauliflower: Remove the leaves and stem from the cauliflower. Cut it into florets.
- Place the florets in a food processor and pulse until they resemble rice grains. Alternatively, grate the florets using a box grater.
- Cook the Vegetables: In a large skillet, heat the olive oil over medium heat.
- Add the finely chopped onion and sauté for 4-5 minutes until it becomes translucent.
- Add the minced garlic, diced carrot, and diced celery. Cook for another 5 minutes until the vegetables are tender.
- Cook the Cauliflower Rice: Add the cauliflower rice to the skillet, stirring to combine with the vegetables.
- Cook for 5-7 minutes, stirring occasionally, until the cauliflower is tender but not mushy.
- Add Peas and Seasonings: Stir in the thawed peas, toasted slivered almonds, dried thyme, and dried oregano.
- Season with salt and pepper to taste.
- Cook for an additional 2-3 minutes until everything is heated through.
- Remove the skillet from heat and stir in the chopped fresh parsley and lemon juice.
- Transfer the cauliflower rice pilaf to a serving dish and serve immediately.

Nutritional Information (per serving):
- Calories: 120 kcal
- Total Fat: 7g
- Saturated Fat: 1g
- Trans Fat: 0g
- Cholesterol: 0mg
- Sodium: 180mg
- Total Carbohydrates: 12g
- Dietary Fiber: 4g
- Sugars: 4g
- Protein: 4g

Sautéed Spinach with Garlic

Serving: 4 servings
Prep Time: 5 minutes
Cook Time: 10 minutes

Ingredients:
- 1 pound fresh spinach leaves, washed and dried
- 2 tablespoons olive oil
- 4 cloves garlic, thinly sliced
- Salt and pepper, to taste
- 1/4 teaspoon red pepper flakes (optional)
- Juice of 1/2 lemon
- Freshly grated Parmesan cheese (optional, for garnish)

Preparation:
- Prepare the Ingredients: Make sure the spinach leaves are thoroughly washed and dried. Use a salad spinner to remove excess water.
- Thinly slice the garlic cloves.
- Heat the Olive Oil: In a large skillet, heat the olive oil over medium heat.
- Add the sliced garlic and sauté for 1-2 minutes until the garlic is fragrant and golden brown, being careful not to burn it.
- Sauté the Spinach: Add the spinach to the skillet in batches, stirring frequently. The spinach will wilt quickly.
- Continue to add more spinach as it wilts down until all the spinach is in the skillet.

- Season with salt, pepper, and red pepper flakes (if using). Stir to combine.
- Finish with Lemon Juice: Once the spinach is wilted and tender, remove the skillet from the heat.
- Squeeze the juice of half a lemon over the spinach and toss to coat evenly.
- Transfer the sautéed spinach to a serving dish.
- If desired, sprinkle with freshly grated Parmesan cheese before serving.

Nutritional Information (per serving):
- Calories: 70 kcal
- Total Fat: 5g
- Saturated Fat: 1g
- Trans Fat: 0g
- Cholesterol: 0mg
- Sodium: 75mg
- Total Carbohydrates: 5g
- Dietary Fiber: 2g
- Sugars: 1g
- Protein: 2g

Tips:
Garlic: Watch the garlic closely while it sautés to prevent it from burning, which can impart a bitter taste.
Spinach: Fresh spinach is recommended for this recipe, but you can use baby spinach for a more tender texture. Lemon Juice: Adding the lemon juice at the end brightens the flavor and adds a refreshing citrus note.

Baked Sweet Potato Fries

Serving: 4 servings
Prep Time: 10 minutes
Cook Time: 25 minutes

Ingredients:
- 2 large sweet potatoes
- 2 tablespoons olive oil
- 1 teaspoon paprika
- 1/2 teaspoon garlic powder
- 1/2 teaspoon ground cumin
- 1/4 teaspoon black pepper
- 1/4 teaspoon salt
- 1/4 teaspoon cayenne pepper (optional)
- Fresh parsley, chopped (for garnish)

Preparation:
- Preheat the Oven: Preheat your oven to 425°F (220°C). Line a baking sheet with parchment paper or lightly grease it with olive oil.
- Prepare the Sweet Potatoes: Peel the sweet potatoes and cut them into 1/4-inch thick fries. Try to keep them as uniform in size as possible to ensure even cooking.
- Season the Fries: In a large bowl, combine the olive oil, paprika, garlic powder, ground cumin, black pepper, salt, and cayenne pepper (if using).
- Add the sweet potato fries to the bowl and toss until they are evenly coated with the seasoning mixture.
- Arrange and Bake: Spread the seasoned sweet potato fries in a single layer on the prepared baking sheet. Make sure they are not overcrowded to ensure they get crispy.
- Bake in the preheated oven for 20-25 minutes, turning them halfway through, until the fries are golden brown and crispy.
- Remove the sweet potato fries from the oven and transfer them to a serving platter.
- Garnish with chopped fresh parsley and serve immediately.

Nutritional Information (per serving):
- Calories: 150 kcal
- Total Fat: 7g
- Saturated Fat: 1g
- Trans Fat: 0g
- Cholesterol: 0mg
- Sodium: 150mg
- Total Carbohydrates: 20g
- Dietary Fiber: 4g
- Sugars: 5g
- Protein: 2g

Tips:
Crispiness: For extra crispiness, you can soak the cut sweet potato fries in cold water for 30 minutes before seasoning them. Be sure to dry them thoroughly before adding the oil and spices.

Even Cooking: Make sure the fries are spread out in a single layer on the baking sheet. If necessary, use two baking sheets to avoid overcrowding.

Steamed Green Beans with Almonds

Serving: 4 servings
Prep Time: 10 minutes
Cook Time: 10 minutes

Ingredients:
- 1 pound fresh green beans, trimmed
- 2 tablespoons olive oil
- 1/4 cup sliced almonds
- 2 cloves garlic, minced
- 1 tablespoon lemon juice
- Salt and pepper, to taste
- 1 tablespoon chopped fresh parsley (optional)

Preparation:
- Prepare the Green Beans: Trim the ends of the green beans and rinse them thoroughly under cold water.
- Steam the Green Beans: Fill a large pot with about 1 inch of water and place a steamer basket inside. Bring the water to a boil over high heat.
- Add the green beans to the steamer basket, cover the pot, and steam for 5-7 minutes, or until the green beans are tender-crisp. Remove from heat and set aside.
- Toast the Almonds: While the green beans are steaming, heat a large skillet over medium heat. Add the sliced almonds and toast them for 2-3 minutes, stirring frequently, until they are golden brown and fragrant. Be careful not to burn them. Remove the almonds from the skillet and set aside.
- Sauté the Garlic: In the same skillet, add the olive oil and minced garlic. Sauté the garlic for about 1 minute, or until it becomes fragrant and golden. Do not let it burn.
- Combine and Season: Add the steamed green beans to the skillet with the garlic. Toss to coat the green beans evenly with the garlic and olive oil.
- Season with salt and pepper to taste and drizzle with lemon juice. Toss again to combine.
- Transfer the green beans to a serving dish. Sprinkle the toasted almonds over the top and garnish with chopped fresh parsley if desired.
- Serve immediately.

Nutritional Information (per serving):
- Calories: 110 kcal
- Total Fat: 7g
- Saturated Fat: 1g
- Trans Fat: 0g
- Cholesterol: 0mg
- Sodium: 150mg
- Total Carbohydrates: 10g
- Dietary Fiber: 4g
- Sugars: 4g
- Protein: 3g

Tips:
Green Beans: For the best texture and flavor, choose fresh, firm green beans. Frozen green beans can be used in a pinch, but fresh is preferred.

QUINOA PILAF WITH HERBS

Serving: 4 servings
Prep Time: 10 minutes
Cook Time: 20 minutes

Ingredients:
- 1 cup quinoa, rinsed
- 2 cups low-sodium vegetable broth
- 1 tablespoon olive oil
- 1 small onion, finely chopped
- 2 cloves garlic, minced
- 1 carrot, finely diced
- 1 celery stalk, finely diced
- 1/4 cup chopped fresh parsley
- 1/4 cup chopped fresh cilantro
- 1 tablespoon fresh thyme leaves (or 1 teaspoon dried thyme)
- Salt and pepper, to taste
- Juice of 1/2 lemon
- 1/4 cup sliced almonds, toasted (optional)

Preparation:
- Prepare the Quinoa: Rinse the quinoa thoroughly under cold water to remove any bitterness.
- Cook the Quinoa: In a medium saucepan, bring the low-sodium vegetable broth to a boil. Add the rinsed quinoa, reduce the heat to low, cover, and simmer for 15 minutes or until the quinoa is tender and has absorbed all the liquid. Remove from heat and let it sit, covered, for 5 minutes. Fluff with a fork.
- Sauté the Vegetables: While the quinoa is cooking, heat the olive oil in a large skillet over medium heat. Add the finely chopped onion and sauté for about 3-4 minutes until it becomes translucent.
- Add the minced garlic, diced carrot, and diced celery. Cook for another 5 minutes, stirring occasionally, until the vegetables are tender.
- Combine and Season: Add the cooked quinoa to the skillet with the sautéed vegetables. Stir to combine.
- Add the chopped fresh parsley, cilantro, and thyme. Season with salt and pepper to taste. Stir in the lemon juice and mix well.
- Toast the Almonds: In a small dry skillet over medium heat, toast the sliced almonds for about 2-3 minutes, stirring frequently, until they are golden brown and fragrant. Be careful not to burn them.
- Transfer the quinoa pilaf to a serving dish. Sprinkle the toasted almonds over the top (if using).
- Serve immediately, garnished with additional fresh herbs if desired.

Nutritional Information (per serving):
- Calories: 180 kcal
- Total Fat: 7g
- Saturated Fat: 1g
- Trans Fat: 0g
- Cholesterol: 0mg

Grilled Asparagus with Lemon

Serving: 4 servings
Prep Time: 5 minutes
Cook Time: 10 minutes

Ingredients:
- 1 pound fresh asparagus, trimmed
- 1 tablespoon olive oil
- 1 lemon, zested and juiced
- 2 cloves garlic, minced
- Salt and pepper, to taste
- 1 tablespoon fresh parsley, chopped (optional)

Preparation:
- Prepare the Asparagus: Rinse the asparagus under cold water and trim the tough ends by bending each stalk until it snaps naturally. Pat them dry with a kitchen towel.
- Season the Asparagus: In a large bowl, toss the asparagus with olive oil, minced garlic, lemon zest, salt, and pepper until evenly coated.
- Grill the Asparagus: Preheat your grill to medium-high heat. If using a grill pan, heat it over medium-high heat until hot.
- Place the asparagus spears on the grill or grill pan in a single layer. Grill for 3-4 minutes per side, turning occasionally, until the asparagus is tender and has grill marks. The exact cooking time may vary depending on the thickness of the asparagus spears.
- Add Lemon Juice: Once the asparagus is grilled, remove it from the heat and transfer it to a serving platter.
- Squeeze the fresh lemon juice over the grilled asparagus and toss gently to coat.
- Garnish with chopped fresh parsley if desired.
- Serve immediately.

Nutritional Information (per serving):
- Calories: 50 kcal
- Total Fat: 3g
- Saturated Fat: 0.5g
- Trans Fat: 0g
- Cholesterol: 0mg
- Sodium: 60mg
- Total Carbohydrates: 5g
- Dietary Fiber: 2g
- Sugars: 2g
- Protein: 2g

Tips:

Grill Prep: Make sure your grill or grill pan is properly preheated to get the best grill marks and flavor.

Garlic: Mince the garlic finely to ensure it spreads evenly and doesn't burn on the grill.

Lemon: Freshly squeezed lemon juice is best for a bright, tangy flavor. Zest the lemon before juicing for ease.

Asparagus: For even cooking, choose asparagus spears of similar thickness.

Roasted Carrots and Parsnips

Serving: 4 servings
Prep Time: 10 minutes
Cook Time: 35 minutes

Ingredients:
- 4 large carrots, peeled and cut into sticks
- 4 large parsnips, peeled and cut into sticks
- 2 tablespoons olive oil
- 1 teaspoon dried thyme
- 1 teaspoon dried rosemary
- 2 cloves garlic, minced
- Salt and pepper, to taste
- 1 tablespoon fresh parsley, chopped (optional)
- Juice of 1/2 lemon (optional)

Preparation:
- Preheat the Oven: Preheat your oven to 400°F (200°C). Line a large baking sheet with parchment paper or lightly grease it with olive oil.
- Prepare the Vegetables: Peel the carrots and parsnips, then cut them into sticks of similar size to ensure even cooking.
- Season the Vegetables: In a large bowl, combine the carrot and parsnip sticks. Add the olive oil, dried thyme, dried rosemary, minced garlic, salt, and pepper. Toss until the vegetables are evenly coated with the seasoning mixture.
- Roast the Vegetables: Spread the seasoned carrot and parsnip sticks in a single layer on the prepared baking sheet. Make sure they are not overcrowded.
- Roast in the preheated oven for 30-35 minutes, turning halfway through, until the vegetables are tender and golden brown on the edges.
- Finish and Serve: Remove the roasted vegetables from the oven and transfer them to a serving dish.
- If desired, sprinkle with chopped fresh parsley and drizzle with lemon juice for added brightness and flavor.
- Serve immediately.

Nutritional Information (per serving):
- Calories: 120 kcal
- Total Fat: 7g
- Saturated Fat: 1g
- Trans Fat: 0g
- Cholesterol: 0mg
- Sodium: 150mg
- Total Carbohydrates: 15g
- Dietary Fiber: 5g
- Sugars: 6g
- Protein: 2g

Tips:

Cut Uniformly: Ensure that the carrot and parsnip sticks are cut uniformly for even roasting.
Garlic: Mince the garlic finely so it spreads evenly and doesn't burn during roast

Stuffed Portobello Mushrooms

Serving: 4 servings
Prep Time: 15 minutes
Cook Time: 25 minutes

Ingredients:
- 4 large portobello mushrooms
- 1 tablespoon olive oil
- 1 small onion, finely chopped
- 2 cloves garlic, minced
- 1 red bell pepper, finely chopped
- 1 cup spinach, chopped
- 1/4 cup sun-dried tomatoes, chopped
- 1/2 cup low-fat mozzarella cheese, shredded
- 1/4 cup grated Parmesan cheese
- 1/2 teaspoon dried oregano
- 1/2 teaspoon dried basil
- Salt and pepper, to taste
- 1 tablespoon fresh parsley, chopped (for garnish)

Preparation:
- Preheat the Oven: Preheat your oven to 375°F (190°C). Line a baking sheet with parchment paper or lightly grease it with olive oil.
- Prepare the Mushrooms: Gently clean the portobello mushrooms with a damp cloth. Remove the stems and scoop out the gills using a spoon to create space for the stuffing.
- Sauté the Vegetables: Heat the olive oil in a large skillet over medium heat. Add the finely chopped onion and cook for about 3-4 minutes until it becomes translucent.
- Add the minced garlic and cook for another minute until fragrant.
- Stir in the chopped red bell pepper and cook for another 3 minutes until it starts to soften.
- Add the chopped spinach and sun-dried tomatoes, cooking until the spinach is wilted. Season with dried oregano, dried basil, salt, and pepper.
- Stuff the Mushrooms: Place the cleaned portobello mushrooms on the prepared baking sheet.
- Evenly divide the vegetable mixture among the mushroom caps, pressing down lightly to pack the filling.
- Sprinkle the shredded mozzarella and grated Parmesan cheese over the top of the stuffed mushrooms.
- Bake: Bake in the preheated oven for 20-25 minutes until the mushrooms are tender and the cheese is melted and golden brown.
- Remove from the oven and let cool for a couple of minutes. Garnish with chopped fresh parsley before serving.

Nutritional Information (per serving):
- Calories: 150 kcal
- Total Fat: 9g
- Saturated Fat: 3g
- Trans Fat: 0g
- Cholesterol: 15mg
- Sodium: 250mg
- Total Carbohydrates: 10g
- Dietary Fiber: 3g
- Sugars: 4g

Zucchini Noodles with Pesto

Serving: 4 servings
Prep Time: 15 minutes
Cook Time: 5 minutes

Ingredients:
- 4 medium zucchinis, spiralized into noodles
- 2 tablespoons olive oil
- 1 cup fresh basil leaves
- 1/4 cup pine nuts
- 2 cloves garlic, minced
- 1/4 cup grated Parmesan cheese (or nutritional yeast for a vegan option)
- 1/4 cup extra-virgin olive oil
- Juice of 1/2 lemon
- Salt and pepper, to taste
- 1/4 cup cherry tomatoes, halved (optional)
- Fresh basil leaves, for garnish

Preparation:
- Prepare the Zucchini Noodles: Using a spiralizer, create noodles from the zucchinis. If you don't have a spiralizer, you can use a julienne peeler or a regular vegetable peeler to create long strips.
- Make the Pesto: In a food processor, combine the fresh basil leaves, pine nuts, minced garlic, and grated Parmesan cheese. Pulse until the ingredients are finely chopped.
- With the food processor running, slowly drizzle in the extra-virgin olive oil until the mixture is smooth and creamy. Add lemon juice, and season with salt and pepper to taste. Pulse a few more times to combine.
- Cook the Zucchini Noodles: Heat 2 tablespoons of olive oil in a large skillet over medium heat. Add the zucchini noodles and sauté for about 2-3 minutes until they are just tender but still have a bit of crunch. Avoid overcooking as zucchini noodles can become watery.
- Combine and Serve: Remove the skillet from heat and toss the cooked zucchini noodles with the prepared pesto until evenly coated.
- Transfer the pesto zucchini noodles to a serving platter. Garnish with halved cherry tomatoes and fresh basil leaves if desired.
- Serve immediately.

Nutritional Information (per serving):
- Calories: 200 kcal
- Total Fat: 18g
- Saturated Fat: 3g
- Trans Fat: 0g
- Cholesterol: 5mg
- Sodium: 150mg
- Total Carbohydrates: 7g
- Dietary Fiber: 2g
- Sugars: 4g
- Protein: 5g

Tips:
Spiralizing: When spiralizing the zucchini, choose medium-sized zucchinis for the best nutritious and satisfying meal.

Chapter 7

Snacks & Appetizers

Snacks and appetizers for diabetic patients are designed to be nutritious, satisfying, and help maintain stable blood sugar levels. They typically include options that are low in carbohydrates, moderate in healthy fats and protein, and high in fiber. Ideal choices often feature fresh fruits and vegetables, lean proteins like chicken or turkey, and healthy fats such as nuts or avocado. These snacks and appetizers are not only delicious but also support overall health and well-being by promoting balanced nutrition and managing blood glucose levels effectively.

Hummus and Veggie Platter

Serving: 4 servings
Prep Time: 10 minutes
Cook Time: 0 minutes

Ingredients:
- 1 cup hummus (store-bought or homemade)
- 2 large carrots, cut into sticks
- 2 large celery stalks, cut into sticks
- 1 medium cucumber, sliced
- 1 bell pepper (red, yellow, or green), sliced
- Cherry tomatoes, for garnish
- Fresh parsley or cilantro, for garnish
- Whole wheat pita bread or whole grain crackers (optional)

Preparation:
- Prepare the Vegetables: Wash and cut the carrots and celery into sticks. Slice the cucumber and bell pepper into thin strips. Arrange them on a serving platter along with cherry tomatoes.
- Serve the Hummus: Place the hummus in a small bowl and place it in the center of the vegetable arrangement on the platter.
- Garnish and Serve: Garnish the hummus and vegetables with fresh parsley or cilantro for added color and flavor.
- Optionally, serve with whole wheat pita bread or whole grain crackers on the side for dipping.

Nutritional Information (per serving, without pita bread or crackers):
- Calories: 150 kcal
- Total Fat: 8g
- Saturated Fat: 1g
- Trans Fat: 0g
- Cholesterol: 0mg
- Sodium: 300mg
- Total Carbohydrates: 16g
- Dietary Fiber: 6g
- Sugars: 3g
- Protein: 6g

Tips:

Hummus Options: Opt for low-sodium or homemade hummus to control salt intake.

Variety of Vegetables: Use a colorful assortment of vegetables to add visual appeal and a variety of nutrients.

Whole Grain Options: Choose whole wheat pita bread or whole grain crackers for added fiber and complex carbohydrates.

Customization: Feel free to add other vegetables such as radishes, broccoli florets, or sugar snap peas based on personal preference.

A Hummus and Veggie Platter is an excellent choice for diabetic patients as it provides a balance of fiber-rich vegetables and protein-packed hummus. This snack is low in carbohydrates, helping to maintain steady blood sugar levels. It's perfect for parties, gatherings, or simply as a nutritious snack option. Enjoy the vibrant colors and flavors while supporting a healthy lifestyle!

Baked Kale Chips

Serving: 4 servings
Prep Time: 10 minutes
Cook Time: 15 minutes

Ingredients:

- 1 bunch kale (about 6-8 cups), washed and dried thoroughly
- 1 tablespoon olive oil
- 1/2 teaspoon garlic powder
- 1/2 teaspoon paprika
- 1/4 teaspoon salt
- 1/4 teaspoon black pepper
- Optional: 1 tablespoon nutritional yeast for added flavor

Preparation:

- Prepare the Kale: Preheat your oven to 350°F (175°C). Line a baking sheet with parchment paper or lightly grease it with olive oil.
- Wash the kale leaves thoroughly under cold water to remove any dirt or residue. Dry them completely using a kitchen towel or salad spinner. Make sure the leaves are dry to ensure crispy kale chips.
- Remove Stems and Tear: Remove the tough stems from the kale leaves by folding each leaf in half and cutting along the stem. Tear the kale into bite-sized pieces.
- Season the Kale: In a large bowl, toss the kale pieces with olive oil until evenly coated. Sprinkle with garlic powder, paprika, salt, and black pepper.

If using, add nutritional yeast for an extra savory flavor.

- Bake the Kale Chips: Spread the seasoned kale pieces in a single layer on the prepared baking sheet. Avoid overcrowding to ensure even baking.
- Bake in the preheated oven for 12-15 minutes, or until the edges are crisp and slightly browned. Keep an eye on them towards the end to prevent burning.
- Cool and Serve: Remove the kale chips from the oven and let them cool on the baking sheet for a few minutes to crisp up further.
- Transfer the baked kale chips to a serving bowl or platter. They are best enjoyed immediately for maximum crispiness.

Nutritional Information (per serving):

- Calories: 50 kcal
- Total Fat: 3g
- Saturated Fat: 0.5g
- Trans Fat: 0g
- Cholesterol: 0mg
- Sodium: 150mg
- Total Carbohydrates: 5g
- Dietary Fiber: 1g
- Sugars: 0g
- Protein: 2g

Tips:

Dry Kale Thoroughly: Moisture can prevent kale chips from crisping up properly, so ensure the leaves are completely dry before baking.

Stuffed Mini Bell Peppers

Serving: 4 servings (about 16 stuffed mini bell peppers)
Prep Time: 20 minutes
Cook Time: 15 minutes

Ingredients:
- 16 mini bell peppers, assorted colors
- 1 cup cooked quinoa
- 1/2 cup black beans, drained and rinsed
- 1/2 cup corn kernels (fresh, canned, or frozen)
- 1/4 cup diced tomatoes
- 1/4 cup diced red onion
- 1/4 cup chopped fresh cilantro
- 1 teaspoon ground cumin
- 1/2 teaspoon chili powder
- Salt and pepper, to taste
- 1/2 cup shredded cheddar cheese (optional)
- Fresh lime wedges, for serving

Preparation:
- Preheat the Oven: Preheat your oven to 375°F (190°C). Line a baking sheet with parchment paper or lightly grease it with olive oil.
- Prepare the Mini Bell Peppers: Cut the tops off the mini bell peppers and remove the seeds and membranes. Rinse them under cold water and pat dry with a paper towel.
- Prepare the Filling: In a large bowl, combine the cooked quinoa, black beans, corn kernels, diced tomatoes, diced red onion, chopped cilantro, ground cumin, chili powder, salt, and pepper. Mix well until all ingredients are evenly distributed.
- Stuff the Bell Peppers: Spoon the quinoa and vegetable mixture into each mini bell pepper until they are filled to the top. If using, sprinkle shredded cheddar cheese on top of each stuffed pepper.
- Bake the Stuffed Peppers: Place the stuffed mini bell peppers on the prepared baking sheet. Bake in the preheated oven for 12-15 minutes, or until the peppers are tender and the filling is heated through.
- Remove from the oven and let cool slightly before serving. Arrange the stuffed mini bell peppers on a serving platter and garnish with fresh lime wedges.

Nutritional Information (per serving, 4 stuffed peppers):
- Calories: 180 kcal
- Total Fat: 4g
- Saturated Fat: 1g
- Trans Fat: 0g
- Cholesterol: 5mg
- Sodium: 250mg
- Total Carbohydrates: 30g
- Dietary Fiber: 6g
- Sugars: 4g
- Protein: 8g

Almond and Cranberry Energy Bites

Serving: Makes about 20 energy bites
Prep Time: 15 minutes
Cook Time: 0 minutes

Ingredients:

- 1 cup rolled oats
- 1/2 cup almond butter (or any nut butter of choice)
- 1/4 cup honey (or maple syrup for a vegan option)
- 1/4 cup almonds, chopped
- 1/4 cup dried cranberries, chopped
- 1 tablespoon chia seeds
- 1/2 teaspoon vanilla extract
- Pinch of salt
- Additional oats or shredded coconut for rolling (optional)

Preparation:

- Prepare the Base: In a large bowl, combine rolled oats, almond butter, honey (or maple syrup), chopped almonds, dried cranberries, chia seeds, vanilla extract, and a pinch of salt. Mix well until all ingredients are evenly distributed.
- Form the Energy Bites: Take about 1 tablespoon of the mixture and roll it between your palms to form a compact ball. If the mixture is too sticky to handle, refrigerate it for 15-30 minutes before rolling.
- Optional: Roll each energy bite in additional rolled oats or shredded coconut for an extra layer of texture and flavor.
- Store or Serve: Place the rolled energy bites on a baking sheet lined with parchment paper. Repeat until all the mixture is used up, making approximately 20 energy bites.
- Refrigerate the energy bites for at least 30 minutes to firm up before serving. Store any leftovers in an airtight container in the refrigerator for up to 1 week.

Nutritional Information (per energy bite):

- Calories: 90 kcal
- Total Fat: 5g
- Saturated Fat: 0.5g
- Trans Fat: 0g
- Cholesterol: 0mg
- Sodium: 15mg
- Total Carbohydrates: 10g
- Dietary Fiber: 2g
- Sugars: 5g
- Protein: 3g

Tips:
Nut Butter Options: Use almond butter, peanut butter, or any nut butter of your choice. Ensure it's natural and without added sugars or oils.
Sweeteners: Adjust the sweetness by adding more or less honey (or maple syrup) based on personal preference.

Greek Yogurt with Fresh Fruit

Serving: 1 serving
Prep Time: 5 minutes
Cook Time: 0 minutes

Ingredients:
- 1/2 cup plain Greek yogurt (low-fat or non-fat)
- 1/2 cup mixed fresh fruits (such as berries, sliced bananas, or diced mango)
- 1 tablespoon chopped nuts (such as almonds, walnuts, or pistachios)
- 1 teaspoon honey or maple syrup (optional, for added sweetness)
- Fresh mint leaves, for garnish (optional)

Preparation:
- Prepare the Yogurt: Spoon the plain Greek yogurt into a serving bowl or dish.
- Prepare the Fresh Fruit: Wash and prepare the fresh fruits as needed. If using berries, rinse them under cold water and pat dry with a paper towel. Slice bananas or dice mango into bite-sized pieces.
- Assemble the Dish: Arrange the mixed fresh fruits on top of the Greek yogurt.
- Sprinkle chopped nuts over the fruits for added crunch and nutrition.
- Optional Sweetener: Drizzle honey or maple syrup over the Greek yogurt and fruits if desired, for a touch of sweetness.
- Garnish and Serve: Garnish with fresh mint leaves for a refreshing finish.
- Serve immediately and enjoy this nutritious and delicious snack.

Nutritional Information:
- Calories: Approximately 150 kcal (depending on fruit and nut choices)
- Total Fat: 5g
- Saturated Fat: 1g
- Trans Fat: 0g
- Cholesterol: 5mg
- Sodium: 40mg
- Total Carbohydrates: 20g
- Dietary Fiber: 3g
- Sugars: 14g
- Protein: 10g

Tips:
Yogurt Options: Opt for plain Greek yogurt to avoid added sugars. Greek yogurt is high in protein and low in carbohydrates, making it an excellent choice for managing blood sugar levels.

Fruit Choices: Use a variety of fresh fruits based on seasonal availability and personal preference. Berries are particularly low in sugar and high in antioxidants.

Nutritional Benefits: This snack provides a balanced combination of protein, healthy fats, and complex carbohydrates, making it a satisfying option that won't cause rapid spikes in blood sugar levels.

Spiced Nuts and Seeds Mix

Serving: 8 servings (about 1/4 cup per serving)
Prep Time: 5 minutes
Cook Time: 10 minutes

Ingredients:

- 1 cup mixed nuts (such as almonds, walnuts, pecans)
- 1/4 cup pumpkin seeds (pepitas)
- 1/4 cup sunflower seeds
- 1 tablespoon olive oil
- 1 tablespoon honey or maple syrup
- 1 teaspoon ground cinnamon
- 1/2 teaspoon ground cumin
- 1/4 teaspoon cayenne pepper (adjust to taste)
- 1/2 teaspoon salt

Preparation:

- Preheat the Oven: Preheat your oven to 350°F (175°C). Line a baking sheet with parchment paper or lightly grease it with olive oil.
- Mix Nuts and Seeds: In a large bowl, combine the mixed nuts, pumpkin seeds, and sunflower seeds.
- Prepare the Spiced Mix: In a small bowl, whisk together olive oil, honey or maple syrup, ground cinnamon, ground cumin, cayenne pepper, and salt until well combined.
- Coat the Nuts and Seeds: Pour the spiced mixture over the nuts and seeds in the large bowl. Toss well to coat evenly.
- Bake the Spiced Nuts and Seeds: Spread the coated nuts and seeds in a single layer on the prepared baking sheet.
- Bake in the preheated oven for 10-12 minutes, stirring halfway through, until golden and fragrant. Keep an eye on them towards the end to prevent burning.
- Cool and Serve: Remove from the oven and let the spiced nuts and seeds mix cool completely on the baking sheet.
- Once cooled, transfer to an airtight container for storage.

Nutritional Information (per serving, about 1/4 cup):

- Calories: 150 kcal
- Total Fat: 12g
- Saturated Fat: 1.5g
- Trans Fat: 0g
- Cholesterol: 0mg
- Sodium: 120mg
- Total Carbohydrates: 9g
- Dietary Fiber: 2g
- Sugars: 4g
- Protein: 5g

Tips:

Customization: Feel free to customize the spiced nuts and seeds mix with your favorite nuts and seeds, such as cashews, peanuts, or sesame seeds.

Cucumber Slices with Tuna Salad

Serving: Makes about 12 cucumber slices
Prep Time: 15 minutes
Cook Time: 0 minutes

Ingredients:

- 1 can (5 oz) tuna, drained
- 2 tablespoons plain Greek yogurt (low-fat or non-fat)
- 1 tablespoon mayonnaise (light or reduced-fat)
- 1 tablespoon lemon juice
- 1 tablespoon finely chopped red onion
- 1 tablespoon chopped fresh dill (or 1 teaspoon dried dill)
- Salt and pepper, to taste
- 1 large cucumber, washed and sliced into rounds
- Fresh dill sprigs, for garnish (optional)

Preparation:

- Prepare the Tuna Salad: In a medium bowl, combine the drained tuna, plain Greek yogurt, mayonnaise, lemon juice, chopped red onion, chopped fresh dill, salt, and pepper. Mix well until all ingredients are evenly incorporated.
- Assemble the Cucumber Slices: Arrange the cucumber slices on a serving platter or plate.
- Top with Tuna Salad: Spoon a small amount of the tuna salad onto each cucumber slice, spreading it evenly.
- Garnish and Serve: Garnish each cucumber slice with a small sprig of fresh dill, if desired, for an extra touch of flavor and presentation.
- Serve Immediately: Serve the cucumber slices with tuna salad immediately as a nutritious and satisfying snack or appetizer.

Nutritional Information (per cucumber slice with tuna salad):

- Calories: Approximately 30 kcal
- Total Fat: 1g
- Saturated Fat: 0.2g
- Trans Fat: 0g
- Cholesterol: 5mg
- Sodium: 70mg
- Total Carbohydrates: 1g
- Dietary Fiber: 0.2g
- Sugars: 0.5g
- Protein: 5g

Tips:

Cucumber Preparation: Ensure the cucumber slices are thick enough to hold the tuna salad without breaking.

Tuna Options: Use canned tuna in water for a lower-fat option, or tuna packed in olive oil for added richness.

Variations: Add diced celery, bell peppers, or pickles to the tuna salad mixture for additional crunch and flavor.

Make-Ahead: Prepare the tuna salad mixture in advance and store it in the refrigerator.

Apple Slices with Peanut Butter

Serving: 2 servings
Prep Time: 5 minutes
Cook Time: 0 minutes

Ingredients:
- 1 medium apple (such as Gala, Fuji, or Honeycrisp)
- 2 tablespoons natural peanut butter (unsweetened)
- Cinnamon, for sprinkling (optional)

Preparation:
- Prepare the Apple: Wash the apple thoroughly under cold water. Core the apple and cut it into thin slices.
- Serve with Peanut Butter: Arrange the apple slices on a serving plate or platter.
- Spread each apple slice with natural peanut butter.
- Optional Garnish: Sprinkle a dash of cinnamon over the apple slices with peanut butter for added flavor (optional).
- Serve Immediately: Serve the apple slices with peanut butter immediately as a quick and nutritious snack.

Nutritional Information (per serving):

- Calories: Approximately 160 kcal
- Total Fat: 10g
- Saturated Fat: 2g
- Trans Fat: 0g
- Cholesterol: 0mg
- Sodium: 80mg
- Total Carbohydrates: 15g
- Dietary Fiber: 3g
- Sugars: 9g
- Protein: 5g

Cook's Tips:

Apple Varieties: Choose your favorite apple variety for this snack. Crisp and sweet apples work well with peanut butter.

Peanut Butter Options: Use natural peanut butter without added sugars or oils for a healthier option.

Optional Additions: Sprinkle with chopped nuts, raisins, or a drizzle of honey for extra sweetness and texture.

Allergy Note: If allergic to peanuts, substitute with almond butter or another nut or seed butter of your choice.

Apple Slices with Peanut Butter is a satisfying and balanced snack option for diabetic patients, providing a mix of carbohydrates, healthy fats, and protein. The natural sweetness of the apple complements the creamy peanut butter, making it a delicious and nutrient-rich choice that helps maintain stable blood sugar levels. Enjoy this quick and easy snack any time of day for a boost of energy and flavor.

Roasted Chickpeas

Serving: 4 servings
Prep Time: 10 minutes
Cook Time: 40 minutes

Ingredients:

- 1 can (15 oz) chickpeas, drained and rinsed
- 1 tablespoon olive oil
- 1 teaspoon smoked paprika
- 1/2 teaspoon garlic powder
- 1/2 teaspoon ground cumin
- 1/4 teaspoon cayenne pepper (optional, for a spicy kick)
- 1/2 teaspoon salt
- 1/4 teaspoon black pepper

Preparation:

- Preheat the Oven: Preheat your oven to 400°F (200°C). Line a baking sheet with parchment paper or lightly grease it.
- Prepare the Chickpeas: Drain and rinse the chickpeas thoroughly. Pat them dry with a paper towel to remove as much moisture as possible. This helps them roast evenly and become crispy.
- Season the Chickpeas: In a medium bowl, toss the dried chickpeas with olive oil, smoked paprika, garlic powder, ground cumin, cayenne pepper (if using), salt, and black pepper. Ensure the chickpeas are evenly coated with the seasoning.
- Roast the Chickpeas: Spread the seasoned chickpeas in a single layer on the prepared baking sheet. Ensure they are not too crowded to allow for even roasting.
- Roast in the preheated oven for 35-40 minutes, shaking the pan halfway through to ensure even cooking. The chickpeas should be golden brown and crispy.
- Cool and Serve: Remove the roasted chickpeas from the oven and let them cool on the baking sheet for a few minutes. They will continue to crisp up as they cool.
- Serve immediately as a crunchy, savory snack or appetizer. Store any leftovers in an airtight container at room temperature for up to 3 days.

Nutritional Information (per serving):

- Calories: 120 kcal
- Total Fat: 5g
- Saturated Fat: 0.5g
- Trans Fat: 0g
- Cholesterol: 0mg
- Sodium: 300mg
- Total Carbohydrates: 15g
- Dietary Fiber: 4g
- Sugars: 1g
- Protein: 5g

Tips:

Drying the Chickpeas: Properly drying the chickpeas is crucial for achieving a crispy texture. Use a clean kitchen towel or paper towel to blot away excess moisture.

Guacamole with Whole Grain Crackers

Serving: 4 servings
Prep Time: 10 minutes
Cook Time: 0 minutes

Ingredients:
- For the Guacamole:
- 2 ripe avocados
- 1 small tomato, diced
- 1/4 cup red onion, finely chopped
- 1 clove garlic, minced
- 1 lime, juiced
- 1/4 cup fresh cilantro, chopped
- 1/2 teaspoon salt
- 1/4 teaspoon black pepper
- 1/4 teaspoon cumin (optional)
- 1 jalapeño, seeded and finely chopped (optional)
- For Serving:
- 1 cup whole grain crackers (approximately 16-20 crackers)

Preparation:
- Prepare the Avocados: Cut the avocados in half, remove the pits, and scoop the flesh into a medium-sized bowl.
- Mash the Avocados: Using a fork or a potato masher, mash the avocados until they reach your desired consistency. Some prefer a chunkier guacamole, while others like it smoother.
- Mix in the Ingredients: Add the diced tomato, finely chopped red onion, minced garlic, lime juice, chopped fresh cilantro, salt, black pepper, and cumin (if using) to the mashed avocados. Mix well to combine all the ingredients.
- If you like a bit of heat, stir in the finely chopped jalapeño.
- Taste and Adjust: Taste the guacamole and adjust the seasoning as needed. You might want to add more salt, lime juice, or cilantro to suit your preference.
- Serve with Whole Grain Crackers: Transfer the guacamole to a serving bowl. Arrange the whole-grain crackers around the bowl for dipping.
- Serve immediately to enjoy the fresh flavors.

Nutritional Information (per serving):
- Calories: Approximately 200 kcal
- Total Fat: 15g
- Saturated Fat: 2g
- Trans Fat: 0g
- Cholesterol: 0mg
- Sodium: 250mg
- Total Carbohydrates: 16g
- Dietary Fiber: 6g
- Sugars: 1g
- Protein: 3g

Tips:
Ripeness of Avocados: Ensure the avocados are ripe for the best texture and flavor. They should yield slightly to gentle pressure.
Storage: If not serving immediately, cover the guacamole with plastic wrap,

Chapter 8

Desserts

Desserts for diabetic patients can be both delicious and health-conscious, focusing on low-sugar, low-carb, and nutrient-dense ingredients. These desserts aim to satisfy sweet cravings without causing significant spikes in blood sugar levels. Often featuring natural sweeteners like stevia or monk fruit, and incorporating whole foods such as fresh fruits, nuts, seeds, and whole grains, these treats offer a balance of flavor and nutrition. Whether it's a creamy yogurt parfait, a rich dark chocolate mousse, or a fruit-based sorbet, diabetic-friendly desserts allow for indulgence while maintaining dietary goals and supporting overall health.

Chia Seed Pudding with Mango

Serving: 4 servings
Prep Time: 10 minutes
Cook Time: None (Chill time: 4 hours or overnight)

Ingredients:
- 1/2 cup chia seeds
- 2 cups unsweetened almond milk (or any plant-based milk of choice)
- 1 teaspoon vanilla extract
- 1 tablespoon maple syrup (optional, for added sweetness)
- 1 ripe mango, peeled, pitted, and diced
- Fresh mint leaves for garnish (optional)

Preparation:
- Mix the Pudding: In a medium bowl, whisk together the chia seeds, unsweetened almond milk, vanilla extract, and maple syrup (if using). Ensure that the chia seeds are evenly distributed and not clumped together.
- Refrigerate: Cover the bowl and refrigerate for at least 4 hours, or overnight. This allows the chia seeds to absorb the liquid and form a pudding-like consistency.
- Prepare the Mango: While the pudding is set, prepare the mango. Peel, pit, and dice the mango into small cubes. Keep it in the refrigerator until ready to serve.
- Assemble and Serve: Once the chia pudding has set, give it a good stir to break up any clumps. Divide the pudding evenly among 4 serving glasses or bowls.
- Top each serving with the diced mango.
- Garnish with fresh mint leaves if desired.

Nutritional Information (per serving):
- Calories: 180 kcal
- Total Fat: 9g
- Saturated Fat: 1g
- Trans Fat: 0g
- Cholesterol: 0mg
- Sodium: 110mg
- Total Carbohydrates: 21g
- Dietary Fiber: 10g
- Sugars: 10g
- Protein: 5g

Tips:
Sweetness: Adjust the sweetness according to your preference. You can skip the maple syrup entirely if you prefer a less sweet dessert or use a sugar substitute if desired.
Milk Alternatives: Any plant-based milk can be used in this recipe, including coconut milk, soy milk, or oat milk, based on your preference.
Fruit Variations: Feel free to substitute mango with other fruits like berries, kiwi, or peaches for variety.
Texture: Stir the chia seed mixture a couple of times during the first hour of refrigeration to ensure even distribution and prevent clumping.
Chia Seed Pudding with Mango is a delightful and healthy dessert, perfect for diabetic patients.

Dark Chocolate and Almond Bark

Serving: 10 servings
Prep Time: 10 minutes
Cook Time: 10 minutes (plus 1 hour for cooling)

Ingredients:

- 8 ounces dark chocolate (70% cocoa or higher), chopped
- 1 cup whole almonds, lightly toasted
- 1/4 cup unsweetened shredded coconut (optional)
- 1/4 teaspoon sea salt
- 1 teaspoon vanilla extract (optional)
- 1 tablespoon coconut oil (optional, for a smoother texture)

Preparation:

- Prepare the Baking Sheet: Line a baking sheet with parchment paper or a silicone baking mat.
- Toast the Almonds: Preheat your oven to 350°F (175°C). Spread the whole almonds on a baking sheet and toast for 5-7 minutes, or until they are lightly golden and fragrant. Let them cool completely.
- Melt the Chocolate: In a double boiler, melt the dark chocolate over simmering water, stirring occasionally until smooth. Alternatively, you can melt the chocolate in the microwave by heating it in 30-second intervals, stirring between each interval until fully melted.
- If using, stir in the coconut oil and vanilla extract until well combined. The coconut oil helps achieve a smoother texture and a shinier finish.
- Combine Ingredients: Once the chocolate is melted and smooth, remove it from the heat. Stir in the toasted almonds until they are evenly coated with chocolate.
- If you're adding shredded coconut, mix it in at this stage as well.
- Spread the Mixture: Pour the chocolate and almond mixture onto the prepared baking sheet. Spread it into an even layer with a spatula, about 1/4-inch thick.
- Sprinkle the sea salt evenly over the top for a delightful contrast with the dark chocolate.
- Cool and Set:
- Allow the chocolate to cool at room temperature until it is set, which usually takes about 1 hour. For faster settings, you can place the baking sheet in the refrigerator for about 20-30 minutes.
- Break into Pieces: Once the chocolate is completely set, break it into irregular pieces. Store the bark in an airtight container at room temperature or in the refrigerator, depending on your preference.

Nutritional Information (per serving):
- Calories: 180 kcal
- Total Fat: 14g
- Saturated Fat: 6g
- Trans Fat: 0g
- Cholesterol: 0mg

Berry Crumble with Oat Topping

Serving: 6 servings
Prep Time: 15 minutes
Cook Time: 30 minutes

Ingredients:

- For the Filling: 2 cups fresh or frozen mixed berries (blueberries, raspberries, strawberries, blackberries)
- 2 tablespoons fresh lemon juice
- 2 tablespoons cornstarch
- 2 tablespoons sugar substitute (such as Stevia or erythritol)
- 1 teaspoon vanilla extract
- For the Oat Topping:
- 1 cup rolled oats
- 1/4 cup almond flour
- 1/4 cup chopped nuts (such as almonds or walnuts)
- 2 tablespoons sugar substitute (such as Stevia or erythritol)
- 1/2 teaspoon ground cinnamon
- 1/4 cup coconut oil, melted
- 1 teaspoon vanilla extract

Preparation:

- Preheat the Oven: Preheat your oven to 350°F (175°C). Grease a 9-inch baking dish with a small amount of coconut oil or non-stick spray.
- Prepare the Berry Filling: In a large bowl, combine the mixed berries, fresh lemon juice, cornstarch, sugar substitute, and vanilla extract. Mix gently to coat the berries evenly with the cornstarch and sweetener.

- Make the Oat Topping:
- In another bowl, combine the rolled oats, almond flour, chopped nuts, sugar substitute, and ground cinnamon. Pour in the melted coconut oil and vanilla extract, stirring until the mixture is well combined and crumbly.
- Assemble the Crumble:
- Spread the berry mixture evenly in the prepared baking dish.
- Sprinkle the oat topping over the berries, making sure it covers the fruit evenly.
- Bake: Bake in the preheated oven for 25-30 minutes, or until the topping is golden brown and the berry filling is bubbly.
- Cool and Serve: Allow the crumble to cool for a few minutes before serving. This will help the filling to set.
- Serve warm, optionally with a dollop of Greek yogurt or a scoop of sugar-free ice cream.

Nutritional Information (per serving):

- Calories: 170 kcal
- Total Fat: 10g
- Saturated Fat: 4g
- Trans Fat: 0g
- Cholesterol: 0mg
- Sodium: 5mg
- Total Carbohydrates: 20g
- Dietary Fiber: 5g
- Sugars: 5g (natural sugars from berries)
- Protein: 3g

Baked Apples with Cinnamon

Serving: 4
Prep Time: 10 minutes
Cook Time: 30 minutes

Ingredients:
- 4 medium apples (Granny Smith, Honeycrisp, or your favorite variety)
- 2 tablespoons melted unsalted butter or coconut oil
- 1/4 cup old-fashioned rolled oats
- 2 tablespoons chopped nuts (walnuts, pecans, or almonds)
- 2 tablespoons raisins or dried cranberries
- 1 teaspoon ground cinnamon
- 1/4 teaspoon ground nutmeg
- 1/4 teaspoon ground ginger
- 2 tablespoons honey or maple syrup
- 1 teaspoon vanilla extract
- 1/2 cup water

Preparation:
- Preheat the Oven: Preheat your oven to 350°F (175°C). Grease a baking dish lightly with butter or coconut oil.
- Prepare the Apples: Wash the apples thoroughly. Using a paring knife or an apple corer, remove the cores from the apples, leaving about 1/2 inch at the bottom to hold the filling. Make the hole wide enough to stuff the filling but ensure the apple remains intact.
- Make the Filling: In a small bowl, combine the melted butter or coconut oil, rolled oats, chopped nuts, raisins or dried cranberries, ground cinnamon, nutmeg, ginger, honey or maple syrup, and vanilla extract. Mix well until all ingredients are evenly coated.
- Stuff the Apples: Evenly divide the filling mixture and stuff it into the hollowed-out center of each apple, packing it lightly.
- Bake the Apples: Place the stuffed apples in the prepared baking dish. Pour 1/2 cup of water into the bottom of the dish to prevent the apples from drying out during baking.
- Cover the dish with aluminum foil and bake in the preheated oven for 20 minutes.
- After 20 minutes, remove the foil and bake for an additional 10 minutes, or until the apples are tender and the filling is golden brown.
- Allow the baked apples to cool slightly before serving. They can be served warm or at room temperature.

Nutritional Information (per serving):
- Calories: 180 kcal
- Total Fat: 7g
- Saturated Fat: 3g
- Trans Fat: 0g
- Cholesterol: 10mg
- Sodium: 5mg
- Total Carbohydrates: 30g
- Dietary Fiber: 5g
- Sugars: 20g
- Protein: 2g

Greek Yogurt with Honey and Nuts

Serving: 4 servings
Prep Time: 5 minutes
Cook Time: None

Ingredients:
2 cups plain Greek yogurt (non-fat or low-fat)
4 tablespoons honey
1/4 cup walnuts, chopped
1/4 cup almonds, chopped
1/4 teaspoon ground cinnamon (optional)
Fresh mint leaves (for garnish, optional)

Preparation:

- Prepare the Ingredients: Measure out 2 cups of plain Greek yogurt and divide it evenly among four serving bowls.
- Add Honey: Drizzle 1 tablespoon of honey over each serving of yogurt. If you prefer a sweeter taste, you can adjust the amount of honey to your liking.
- Add Nuts: Sprinkle 1 tablespoon each of chopped walnuts and almonds over the top of each serving. Nuts add a delightful crunch and are packed with healthy fats and protein.
- Add Cinnamon (Optional): For an extra touch of flavor, sprinkle a pinch of ground cinnamon over each serving. Cinnamon adds warmth and enhances the natural sweetness of the honey and yogurt.
- Garnish (Optional): If desired, garnish each bowl with a fresh mint leaf for a pop of color and a refreshing hint of mint.
- Serve: Serve immediately or refrigerate for up to an hour if you prefer it chilled. Enjoy this simple and nutritious dessert that is both satisfying and delicious.

Nutritional Information (per serving):
- Calories: 180 kcal
- Total Fat: 8g
- Saturated Fat: 1g
- Trans Fat: 0g
- Cholesterol: 5mg
- Sodium: 50mg
- Total Carbohydrates: 22g
- Dietary Fiber: 2g
- Sugars: 18g
- Protein: 8g

Tips:
Greek Yogurt: Choose plain Greek yogurt to avoid added sugars and keep the recipe diabetes-friendly. Non-fat or low-fat options are best.
Honey: Use raw honey for its natural antioxidants and better flavor. Adjust the amount of honey based on your sweetness preference.
Nuts: Feel free to substitute walnuts and almonds with other nuts like pistachios or pecans if desired.
Cinnamon: Adding a pinch of cinnamon not only enhances the flavor but may also help in regulating blood sugar levels.

Coconut Flour Cookies

Serving: 12 cookies
Prep Time: 10 minutes
Cook Time: 15 minutes

Ingredients:

- 1/2 cup coconut flour
- 1/4 cup coconut oil, melted
- 1/4 cup honey or a low-glycemic sweetener like erythritol
- 1/4 teaspoon salt
- 1/2 teaspoon baking soda
- 1/2 teaspoon vanilla extract
- 2 large eggs
- 1/4 cup dark chocolate chips (optional)

Preparation:

- Preheat the Oven: Preheat your oven to 350°F (175°C). Line a baking sheet with parchment paper.
- Mix the Dry Ingredients: In a medium-sized bowl, whisk together the coconut flour, salt, and baking soda until well combined.
- Combine Wet Ingredients: In another bowl, mix the melted coconut oil, honey (or low-glycemic sweetener), vanilla extract, and eggs. Beat until smooth and well blended.
- Combine Wet and Dry Ingredients: Gradually add the dry ingredients to the wet mixture, stirring until a dough forms. If using, fold in the dark chocolate chips.

- Shape the Cookies: Scoop out small amounts of dough (about 1 tablespoon each) and roll them into balls. Place the dough balls on the prepared baking sheet, flattening them slightly with your palm or the back of a spoon.
- Bake: Bake in the preheated oven for 12-15 minutes, or until the edges are golden brown. The cookies will be soft when you take them out of the oven but will firm up as they cool.
- Cool and Serve: Allow the cookies to cool on the baking sheet for 5 minutes before transferring them to a wire rack to cool completely. Enjoy these delicious, diabetic-friendly treats!

Nutritional Information (per serving):

- Calories: 100 kcal
- Total Fat: 7g
- Saturated Fat: 5g
- Trans Fat: 0g
- Cholesterol: 25mg
- Sodium: 60mg
- Total Carbohydrates: 8g
- Dietary Fiber: 3g
- Sugars: 4g
- Protein: 2g

Tips:

Coconut Flour: Coconut flour absorbs a lot of moisture, so it's important to follow the recipe closely. Substituting it with other flours will not yield the same results.

Frozen Banana Bites

Serving: 4 servings
Prep Time: 10 minutes (plus 2 hours freezing time)
Cook Time: 0 minutes

Ingredients:

- 2 ripe bananas
- 1/2 cup dark chocolate chips (70% cocoa or higher)
- 1 tablespoon coconut oil
- 1/4 cup chopped nuts (such as almonds, walnuts, or peanuts)
- 1/4 cup unsweetened shredded coconut (optional)

Preparation:

- Prepare the Bananas: Peel the bananas and cut them into 1-inch thick slices.
- Arrange and Freeze: Place the banana slices on a parchment-lined baking sheet in a single layer. Make sure they are not touching each other to prevent sticking.
- Freeze the banana slices for at least 1 hour or until they are firm.
- Prepare the Chocolate Coating: In a microwave-safe bowl, combine the dark chocolate chips and coconut oil.
- Microwave in 30-second intervals, stirring after each interval, until the chocolate is completely melted and smooth.
- Coat the Banana Slices: Remove the frozen banana slices from the freezer.

- Using a fork or toothpick, dip each banana slice into the melted chocolate, ensuring it is fully coated. Allow any excess chocolate to drip off.
- Place the chocolate-coated banana slices back onto the parchment-lined baking sheet.
- Add Toppings: Before the chocolate sets, sprinkle the coated banana slices with chopped nuts and unsweetened shredded coconut (if using).
- Freeze Again: Return the baking sheet to the freezer and freeze the banana bites for another hour or until the chocolate is fully set.
- Serve: Once frozen solid, transfer the banana bites to an airtight container or zip-lock bag for storage.
- Serve directly from the freezer for a refreshing, sweet treat.

Nutritional Information (per serving):

- Calories: 140 kcal
- Total Fat: 9g
- Saturated Fat: 5g
- Trans Fat: 0g
- Cholesterol: 0mg
- Sodium: 5mg
- Total Carbohydrates: 16g
- Dietary Fiber: 3g
- Sugars: 9g
- Protein: 2g

Pumpkin Pie Smoothie

Serving: 2 servings
Prep Time: 5 minutes
Cook Time: 0 minutes

Ingredients:

- 1 cup unsweetened almond milk
- 1/2 cup canned pumpkin puree
- 1 ripe banana, frozen
- 1/2 teaspoon ground cinnamon
- 1/4 teaspoon ground nutmeg
- 1/4 teaspoon ground ginger
- 1/4 teaspoon vanilla extract
- 1 tablespoon chia seeds (optional)
- 1 tablespoon honey or maple syrup (optional, adjust to taste)
- Ice cubes (optional, for a colder smoothie)

Preparation:

- Combine Ingredients: In a blender, combine the unsweetened almond milk, canned pumpkin puree, frozen banana, ground cinnamon, ground nutmeg, ground ginger, vanilla extract, and chia seeds (if using).
- Blend Until Smooth: Blend on high speed until all ingredients are well combined and the mixture is smooth. If you prefer a thicker smoothie, add more ice cubes and blend again.
- Adjust Sweetness: Taste the smoothie and add honey or maple syrup if desired, adjusting to your preferred level of sweetness.
- Serve: Pour the pumpkin pie smoothie into glasses.
- Optionally, sprinkle a dash of cinnamon on top for garnish.

Nutritional Information (per serving):

- Calories: 120 kcal
- Total Fat: 2g
- Saturated Fat: 0g
- Trans Fat: 0g
- Cholesterol: 0mg
- Sodium: 90mg
- Total Carbohydrates: 27g
- Dictary Fiber: 6g
- Sugars: 12g
- Protein: 2g

Tips:

Frozen Banana: Using a frozen banana adds creaminess to the smoothie without the need for ice.

Spices: Adjust the amount of cinnamon, nutmeg, and ginger according to your taste preferences.

Chia Seeds: Chia seeds add fiber and can help thicken the smoothie. They also provide omega-3 fatty acids.

Sweeteners: If you prefer a sweeter smoothie, add more honey or maple syrup, or use sweetened almond milk.

Avocado Chocolate Mousse

Serving: 4 servings
Prep Time: 10 minutes
Cook Time: 0 minutes

Ingredients:

- 2 ripe avocados
- 1/4 cup unsweetened cocoa powder
- 1/4 cup milk (or dairy-free alternative)
- 1/4 cup honey or maple syrup (adjust to taste)
- 1 teaspoon vanilla extract
- Pinch of salt
- Fresh berries or mint leaves, for garnish (optional)

Preparation:

- Prepare the Avocados: Cut the avocados in half, remove the pit, and scoop out the flesh into a blender or food processor.
- Blend the Ingredients: Add cocoa powder, milk, honey or maple syrup, vanilla extract, and a pinch of salt to the blender with the avocado.
- Blend on high until the mixture is smooth and creamy, scraping down the sides of the blender as needed to ensure everything is well combined.
- Adjust Sweetness: Taste the mousse and adjust sweetness as desired by adding more honey or maple syrup if needed.
- Chill (Optional):For a firmer texture, chill the mousse in the refrigerator for at least 30 minutes before serving.
- Divide the avocado chocolate mousse into serving dishes.
- Garnish with fresh berries or mint leaves if desired.

Nutritional Information (per serving):

- Calories: 200 kcal
- Total Fat: 14g
- Saturated Fat: 2g
- Trans Fat: 0g
- Cholesterol: 0mg
- Sodium: 50mg
- Total Carbohydrates: 20g
- Dietary Fiber: 8g
- Sugars: 10g
- Protein: 3g

Tips:

Avocado Ripeness: Ensure the avocados are ripe for a smoother texture.

Sweetener Options: Use honey or maple syrup as natural sweeteners, adjusting to taste.

Texture: Blend the mousse thoroughly to achieve a silky-smooth consistency.

Garnish: Fresh berries or mint leaves add a refreshing contrast to the rich chocolate flavor.

Avocado Chocolate Mousse is a delightful dessert option for diabetic patients, offering a creamy texture with the health benefits of avocados. It's rich in fiber, healthy fats, and antioxidants, making it a guilt-free indulgence.

Raspberry Sorbet

Serving: About 4 servings
Prep Time: 10 minutes
Cook Time: 0 minutes

Ingredients:
- 4 cups fresh or frozen raspberries
- 1/2 cup water
- 1/4 cup honey or maple syrup (adjust to taste)
- 1 tablespoon fresh lemon juice
- Fresh mint leaves, for garnish (optional)

Preparation:

- Prepare the Raspberries: If using fresh raspberries, rinse them thoroughly under cold water and pat dry with a paper towel. If using frozen raspberries, thaw them slightly.
- Blend the Ingredients: In a blender or food processor, combine the raspberries, water, honey or maple syrup, and fresh lemon juice.
- Blend until smooth and creamy. Taste and adjust sweetness with more honey or maple syrup if desired.
- Strain (optional): For a smoother texture, you can strain the raspberry mixture through a fine mesh sieve to remove the seeds. Press down with a spoon to extract as much liquid as possible.
- Chill: Transfer the raspberry mixture to a shallow dish or baking pan. Cover and place in the freezer for about 2-3 hours, stirring every 30 minutes with a fork to break up ice crystals, until the sorbet is firm but scoopable.
- Scoop the raspberry sorbet into bowls or glasses. Garnish with fresh mint leaves if desired.
- Serve immediately as a refreshing dessert.

Nutritional Information (per serving):
- Calories: 100 kcal
- Total Fat: 1g
- Saturated Fat: 0g
- Trans Fat: 0g
- Cholesterol: 0mg
- Sodium: 0mg
- Total Carbohydrates: 25g
- Dietary Fiber: 8g
- Sugars: 17g
- Protein: 2g

Tips:

Sweetness: Adjust the sweetness of the sorbet to your preference. Raspberries can vary in tartness, so taste the mixture before freezing and add more sweetener if needed.

Texture: Stirring the sorbet mixture frequently while freezing helps to achieve a smoother texture. Breaking up the ice crystals ensures a light and fluffy consistency.

Variations: You can substitute raspberries with other berries such as strawberries or blackberries for different flavors of sorbet.

Stora

14 DAYS MEAL PLAN

Day 1:
- **Breakfast:** Greek Yogurt Parfait with Berries
- **Lunch:** Chicken and Broccoli Casserole
- **Dinner:** Grilled Asparagus with Lemon

Day 2:
- **Breakfast:** Spinach and Mushroom Omelette
- **Lunch:** Stuffed Portobello Mushrooms
- **Dinner:** Baked Cod with Asparagus

Day 3:
- **Breakfast:** Quinoa Breakfast Bowl with Almonds and Berries
- **Lunch:** Turkey Meatballs with Zucchini Noodles
- **Dinner:** Roasted Carrots and Parsnips

Day 4:
- **Breakfast:** Overnight Chia Seed Pudding with Fresh Fruit
- **Lunch:** Shrimp and Avocado Tacos
- **Dinner:** Spaghetti Squash with Tomato Sauce

Day 5:
- **Breakfast:** Scrambled Eggs with Sautéed Spinach and Garlic
- **Lunch:** Cauliflower Rice Pilaf with Herbs
- **Dinner:** Garlic Roasted Brussels Sprouts

Day 6:
- **Breakfast:** Smoothie with Spinach, Berries, and Protein Powder
- **Lunch:** Stuffed Portobello Mushrooms
- **Dinner:** Grilled Asparagus with Lemon

Day 7:
- **Breakfast:** Greek Yogurt Parfait with Berries
- **Lunch:** Turkey Meatballs with Zucchini Noodles
- **Dinner:** Baked Cod with Asparagus

Day 8:
- **Breakfast:** Spinach and Mushroom Omelette
- **Lunch:** Quinoa Pilaf with Herbs
- **Dinner:** Roasted Carrots and Parsnips

Day 9:
- **Breakfast:** Quinoa Breakfast Bowl with Almonds and Berries
- **Lunch:** Chicken and Broccoli Casserole
- **Dinner:** Spaghetti Squash with Tomato Sauce

Day 10:
- **Breakfast:** Overnight Chia Seed Pudding with Fresh Fruit
- **Lunch:** Shrimp and Avocado Tacos
- **Dinner:** Garlic Roasted Brussels Sprouts

Day 11:
- **Breakfast:** Scrambled Eggs with Sautéed Spinach and Garlic
- **Lunch:** Cauliflower Rice Pilaf with Herbs
- **Dinner:** Grilled Asparagus with Lemon

Day 12:
- **Breakfast:** Smoothie with Spinach, Berries, and Protein Powder
- **Lunch:** Stuffed Portobello Mushrooms
- **Dinner:** Baked Cod with Asparagus

Day 13:
- **Breakfast:** Greek Yogurt Parfait with Berries
- **Lunch:** Turkey Meatballs with Zucchini Noodles
- **Dinner:** Quinoa Pilaf with Herbs

Day 14:
- **Breakfast:** Spinach and Mushroom Omelette
- **Lunch:** Chicken and Broccoli Casserole
- **Dinner:** Roasted Carrots and Parsnips

This 14-day ensures balanced meals that support stable blood sugar levels and overall health. Adjust portion sizes and specific ingredients based on individual dietary needs and preferences. Regularly monitor blood sugar levels and consult with a healthcare professional for personalized guidance on managing diabetes through diet.

TIPS FOR LONG-TERM SUCCESS

- **Regular Monitoring:** Consistently monitor blood sugar levels as advised by your healthcare provider. This helps track progress and adjust management strategies accordingly.
- **Healthy Eating:** Follow a balanced diet rich in fruits, vegetables, whole grains, lean proteins, and healthy fats. Limit processed foods, sugars, and saturated fats to help manage blood sugar levels and maintain overall health.
- **Physical Activity:** Incorporate regular exercise into your routine, aiming for at least 150 minutes of moderate-intensity aerobic activity per week, along with muscle-strengthening exercises.
- **Medication Adherence:** Take prescribed medications as directed by your healthcare team to effectively manage blood sugar levels and prevent complications.
- **Stress Management:** Practice stress-reduction techniques such as deep breathing, meditation, yoga, or hobbies to manage stress levels, which can affect blood sugar control.
- **Regular Check-**ups: Attend regular medical check-ups, including eye exams, foot exams, and dental exams, to detect and address any potential complications early.
- **Education and Support:** Stay informed about diabetes management through education programs, support groups, or counseling. Knowledge empowers you to make informed decisions about your health.
- **Hydration:** Drink plenty of water throughout the day to stay hydrated, which supports overall health and can aid in managing blood sugar levels.
- **Sleep**: Prioritize good sleep hygiene to ensure adequate rest. Poor sleep can affect blood sugar control and overall well-being.
- **Lifestyle Modifications:** Make sustainable lifestyle changes, such as quitting smoking if applicable, to further support your overall health and diabetes management goals.

By adopting these tips and working closely with your healthcare team, you can promote long-term success in managing diabetes and leading a healthy, fulfilling life.